PHARMACOLOGY - RESEARCH, SAFETY TESTING AND REGULATION

HANDBOOK OF NOVEL DRUG DELIVERY

Pharmacology - Research, Safety Testing and Regulation

Additional books and e-books in this series can be found on Nova's website under the Series tab.

PHARMACOLOGY - RESEARCH, SAFETY TESTING AND REGULATION

HANDBOOK OF NOVEL DRUG DELIVERY

BALRAM AMBADE
RAJENDRA KUMAR JANGDE
AND
SULEKHA KHUTE

nova
science publishers
New York

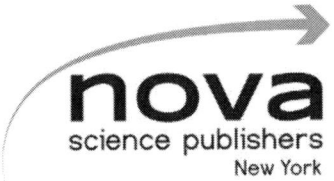

Library of Congress Cataloging-in-Publication Data

Names: Ambade, Balram, author.
Title: Handbook of novel drug delivery / Balram Ambade, Rajendra Kumar Jangde, Sulekha Khute.
Description: New York : Nova Science Publishers, [2021] | Series: Pharmacology - research, safety testing and regulation | Includes bibliographical references and index. |
Identifiers: LCCN 2020056057 (print) | LCCN 2020056058 (ebook) | ISBN 9781536190755 (paperback) | ISBN 9781536190915 (adobe pdf)
Subjects: LCSH: Drug delivery systems.
Classification: LCC RS199.5 .A43 2021 (print) | LCC RS199.5 (ebook) | DDC 615/.6--dc23
LC record available at https://lccn.loc.gov/2020056057
LC ebook record available at https://lccn.loc.gov/2020056058

Published by Nova Science Publishers, Inc. † New York

CONTENTS

PREFACE

This book advances in the field of novel drug delivery having exposure of novel molecules with the potential to transform the treatment and preclusion of wound healing. However, such potential is severely compromised by significant obstacles to delivery of these drugs *in vivo*. Sophisticated drug delivery and targeting can offer significant advantages to conventional drugs, such as increased efficiency, handiness, and the potential for line extensions and market expansion. It is a simple accessible and easy-to-read handbook, Drug Delivery and Targeting for Pharmacists and Pharmaceutical Scientists is the first book to provide a comprehensive introduction to the principles of advanced drug delivery system.

Chapter 1

WOUND HEALING

1. INTRODUCTION

1.1. Wound

A wound as a defect or an end in the skin results from the material and thermal break that deteriorate physiological condition [1]. An injury is outlined as damage or disruption to the usual anatomical constitution and function. The superficial damage in the dermis' epithelial integrity may be more profound, extending into subcutaneous tissue with injury to different structures similar to tendons, muscle groups, vessels, nerves, parenchymal organs, and even bone [2-3]. According to wound curing high society, "a wound is an effect of 'disruption of standard anatomic put together and function.' Additionally, there are variations between tissues in terms of the time required for complete regeneration. Wound healing time may also be numerous, and some wounds may take up to a year or extra to heal entirely [4-6]. A thoroughly healed wound is defined as one who has been lower back to an anatomical structure, operate and look of the tissue within a cheap period. More often than not, most injuries are the effect of straightforward accidents; however, some wounds do not heal in a well-timed and orderly method. Multiple systemic and neighborhood reasons may sluggish the course of wound treatment by inflicting disturbances in the finely balanced restore approaches, leading to continual non-medication wound.

Wound healing is a composite and dynamic process in which skin and tissue repair themselves after injury. Wound healing is a damaged area of an emotional body process in which skin and tissue under it improve themselves after injury. Wound healing depends on each patient's needs and depends on several factors. If any injury damages its barrier, a various biological event occurs to repair the damage. It begins to epidermal layer and might take years.

1.2. Types of Wounds

1.2.1. Acute Wounds

These are commonly handkerchief injuries that cure entirely, within the reasonable time frame, usually 8-12 weeks [7]. The major causes of acute wounds embrace cuts and tears caused by a friction connection between skin and fast surfaces. For example, the operation to cast off a gentle tissue tumor located in the dermis and underlying parenchymal can frequently outcomes in a tremendous albeit noncom-contaminated wound that can't be healed by way of predominant intention due to the colossal defect within the tissue. Aggravating damages are additionally customarily encountered. They could also be involved in the delicate tissues or related to bone fractures [8]. A horrendous injury is ordered regardless of whether it is clean or chaotic. A surgical wound is either chiseled and suture or exposed to mend by a specialist. The damage breaks the trustworthiness of the skin, including the epidermis and dermis. Surgical injuries are ordered in connection to the potential for disease in the wound: they are thought to be either perfect, clean sullied, tainted, or grimy. Surgical injuries that are polluted or contaminated are left open post-surgery while the disease resolves, and after that, they are sutured shut. Premature essential conclusions on these occasions can be adverse to a fruitful result. Administration of a horrible extreme injury at first includes crisis strategies, revival, and dissemination to the partial appendage. The blood supply must be improved, any necrotic tissue debridement away as this can go about as a point of convergence for microorganisms and the injury flooded. Antimicrobials and lockjaw are typically given prophylactically.

1.2.2. Chronic Wounds

On the other way, it comes out from several tissue damages that healed slowly; it does not heal beyond two weeks and, in general, reoccur [9]. Such wounds fail to heal due to repeated injuries, insults, or underlying physiological conditions reminiscent of diabetes and malignancies, chronic infection, poor significant Healing, and other patient-related factors [10]. This outcome disrupts the systematic and well-synchronized pursuits for the wound therapy process [11]. A steady-state of inflammation in the wound creates a cascade of tissue responses that collectively cause to endure a non-rehabilitation state. Because the medications proceed in an uncoordinated manner, wise and anatomical results are negative, and these wounds almost always relapse [12].

2. Wound Healing

Wound remedy progresses using a series of mutual dependence and overlapping stages. A kind of cellular and matrix add-ons act together to reestablish the wholeness of damaged tissues and substitute. The misplaced tissue and tissue repair process and wound healing phase are mentioned in Figures 1 and 2 [13]. Separate parts of wounds may be at extraordinary stages of treatment at any one time [14]. Timing and interaction between the accessories taking part in the wound remedy system range for acute and chronic wounds, even though the main phases stay identical [15]. Natural wound therapy is a dynamic series of movements involving the coordinated interplay of blood cells, proteins, proteases, growth causes, and extracellular matrix accessories.

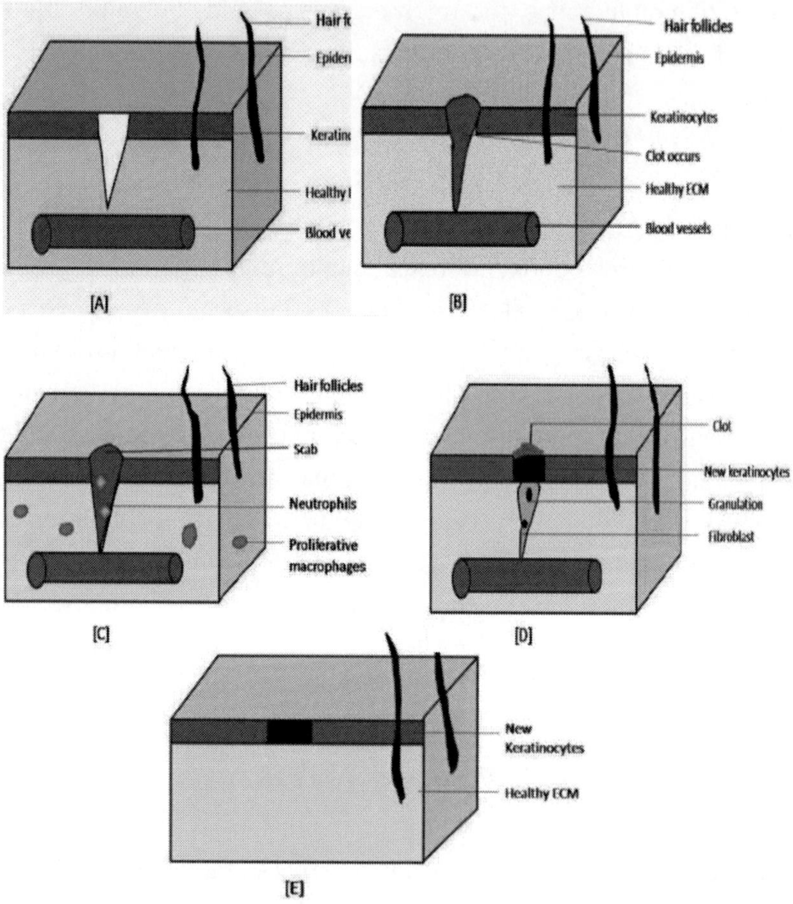
[A]
Hair follicles
Epidermis
Keratinocytes
Clot occurs
Healthy ECM
Blood vessels
[B]
Hair follicles
Epidermis
Scab
Neutrophils
Proliferative macrophages
[C]
Clot
New keratinocytes
Granulation
Fibroblast
[D]
New Keratinocytes
Healthy ECM
[E]

Figure 1. [A] Wound Rapid [B] Hemostasis [C] Inflammation [D] Proliferation [E] Maturation.

2.1. Description of Phases

2.1.1. Hemostasis and Inflammation

The inflammatory phase is characterized by hemostasis and inflammation. Bleeding occurs when the dermis is damaged and serves to flush out micro-organism and antigens from the wound. Moreover, bleeding activates hemostasis initiated by exudates accessories reminiscent of clotting motives [16]. After damage occurs, the mobile phone membranes liberate the influential familiar instructor's thromboxane A2 and prostaglandin 2-alpha [17]. The clotting mechanism resulting in coagulation of the exudates and conjugation with fibrin community formation, produces a clot and stops bleeding. The clot dries to a kind of scab and presents force and aid to the injured tissues. Hemostasis plays a vital role in wound treatment. The inflammatory phase happens close to the same time as hemostasis. Within a couple of minutes of injury to 24 hr and last for approximately three days. They open of protein well off exudates into the injury reasons, vasodilatation. Methods for the arrival of histamine and serotonin enables phagocytes to enter the injury and inundate futile cells. Hard necrotic tissue is liquefied by an enzymatic motion to provide a yellowish colored mass described as slightly. Platelets liberated from broken blood vessels come to be activated as they come into contact with mature collagen and kind aggregates as a part of the clotting mechanism.

2.1.2. Migratory and Proliferative Phase

It promotes the locomotive property of epithelial cells and fibroblasts to the injured area and replaces the damaged and unbound tissue. These cells live new and more vigorous life to the margins, firstly forming overwound under a dries scab convoy with an epithelial thickening. In this reepithelization, it approximately takes 3-10 days. The therapy approach's main focus lies in protecting the wound surfaces, forming granulation tissue, and restoring the vascular community. For this reason, next to the immigration of regional fibroblasts along with the fibrin network. The starting of re-epithelization from the wound edges, revascularization, and angiogenesis get activated [18]. Below the manipulate of regulating cytokines, the synthesis of collagen, fibronectin, and other standard supplies needed for wound medication by way of fibroblasts represent the foundation for the brand new matrix of connective tissue, serving for the closure of tissue gaps and the restoration of the mechanical strength of the wound. Therefore, the collagen synthesis increases for the damage, even as fibroblasts' proliferation declines successively, adjusting stability between synthesis and degradation of extracellular matrix (ECM). This method is activated via signaling pathways of epithelial and non-epithelial cells on the wound edges, unlocking many exceptional cytokines and growth reasons. Moreover, the abolition of the contact inhibition and physical anxiety desmosomes hemidesmosomes produces lipid mediators. It activates membrane – related kinases resulting in increased permeability of the ions' membrane, e.g., calcium. This shows an initiating signal to cells on the wound edges with a retraction and reorganization of their intracellular tonofilaments within the course of migration [19].

2.1.3. Remodeling

Remodeling is the last section of wound healing and occurs from day 21 to 1 year after damage. The formation of granulation tissues stops via apoptosis of the cells. A mature wound is, as a consequence, characterized as vascular and cellular. For the period of the maturation of damage, the add-ons of the ECM bear notable changes. Collagen 3, which used to be produced within the proliferative section, is replaced with the more suitable collagen. This form of collagen is oriented in small parallel bundles and is consequently different from the basket weave collagen in the healthy dermis. In a while, myofibroblasts motivate wound contractions through couple attachment to collagen and help reduce the outside of the establishing scar [20].

3. Wound Debridement

It's main to cast off necrotic tissue or international material from areas around the wound to develop wound treatment probabilities, and this procedure is often called wound debridement. Debridement is the essential role play in the open wound mattress can't be revealed and assessed efficiently with necrotic tissue. The presence of necrotic tissue or overseas fabric in a wound also raises the danger of illness and sepsis and prolongs the inflammatory segment, inhibiting wound Healing. Several ways are utilized for wound debridement are surgical tools with scissors, hydrotherapy, wound water system, and autolysis disposal. For example, making utilization of hydrogen dressings, enzymatic using bacterial determined collagenase or guideline streptokinase. In addition to casting off necrotic tissue, maggots disinfect wound by killing microorganisms and stimulating turbo wound treatment exceptionally for chronic wounds. It has been recommended that maggots also enable the construction of granulation tissue [21].

4. Approaches for Wound Healing

A large number of new technologies available for burns and wound care. Silver dressings are time-honoured in burn and wound care; however, new forms of delivery purpose to increase the efficacy while minimizing facet effects. Harmful strain wound gadgets are relatively new in wound care healing, and their signs are continually expanding to encompass aspects of wound administration that previously had only a few options. Developed wound dressings product can aid alter the wound environment to optimize remedy conditions. With the appearance of biosynthesis and tissue engineering and epidermis, a substitute is being created that no longer best provides novel robust temporary protection of wounds and changes the wound management paradigm [22].

4.1. Silver

Using silver to avoid and deal with the infection is probably the earliest type of wound care, documented as early as 69BC, and one of the spirited brand new technologies within the realm of antimicrobial prophylaxis. Because silver does have this sort of favourable broad spectrum insurance policy, primarily in antibiotics resistant organisms, with little considerable toxicity. Quantities of new silver-containing wound commodities develop to capitalize on its wound remedy advantage, even tailoring the delivery to the most potent approach with the side effects. Nanocrystalline silver dressings were created and delivered in the late 1990s and are the most recent silver injury dressing type. These items have been intended to conquer a portion of the misconduct of past silver dressings. The standard products currently in use include two layers of high-density polyethene web sandwiching, a rayon/polyester gauze layer. The outer layer is coated with nanocrystalline, a non charged form of silver, and the inside layer helps preserve a moist environment for wound remedy. Lastly, silver is an effective form of sensory perception for preventing or treating infection over a large amount of microflora with numerous side effects. It is useful, as antibiotic-resistant micro-organisms [23].

4.2. Negative Pressure Wound Devices

Advances devices comprise smaller size, enabling transportable items for home use, increased ability to put off massive quantities of fluid. The ability to instil fluids within the wound for regular irrigation, refinements in the foam with extra constant pore sizes, unique sponge substances together with silver, and high security and alarm techniques [24]. Acute wounds are extra often being dealt with with Negative pressure wound device (NPWD) closure. In patients with huge comorbidities or other serious mishaps, NPWDs can be used in immense delicate tissue wounds, tainted injuries, and wounds with bargained tissues. In a perfect world, fragile or muscles must be put between the constitution and the wipe, yet Vaseline or silicone work must be utilized when this isn't suitable. The forces give impermanent scope and additional instruments to the expulsion of intra abdominal sickness. These patients most likely required giant hernia repairs with mesh; however, with the NPWD, a high percentage are capable of being, in particular, closed [25-26].

5. Advanced Dressings

The system of autolysis is critical in wound care and advanced wound dressing material mentioned in Table 1. If occlusive dressing is outfitted as a boundary to the outside climate. Physical make-up has phagocytes variables. These items extend from occlusive movies comparing to Tega-derm, impervious to liquid, and microorganism. Additionally, turbo remedy occasions from advanced dressings imply an overall lowered therapy of interval [27].

Table 1. Phases of wound healing

Phase	Duration	Important physiological activity
Hemostasis	Immediate	Formation of the fibrin clot and platelet plug. Vasoconstriction of injured skin or soft tissue.
Inflammation	One day – 2 weeks	Leucocyte recruitment, neutrophil infiltration, secretion of pro-inflammatory cytokines, growth factors, and reactive oxygen species.
Proliferation	Two days – 3 weeks	Fibroblast proliferation, collagen synthesis, angiogenesis, and formation of granulation tissue.
Maturation	Three weeks – 2 years	Re-epithelialisation, the formation of myofibroblasts, collagen remodeling, and scar tissue formation.

5.1. Gauze Dressings

Gauze dressings are created from woven and non-woven fibres of cotton, rayon polyester, or a combo of each. Using soaked gauze for packing open surgical and cavity wounds has also been reviewed within the gentle of their known shortcomings in evaluating the extra recent dressings presently on hand for power wounds. Sterile gauze pads are used to pack open wounds to take in fluid and exudate with the sauce's fibres, acting as a filter to draw fluid far away from the scars. It's misplaced cost mighty when compared with the extra ultra-modern dressings. Although gauze dressings can furnish some bacterial defence, this is misplaced when the sauces' outer surface becomes moistened both by wound exudates or external fluids. Furthermore, gauze dressings are likely to be aware that adherent to wounds as fluid construction diminishes and is painful to do away with, causing sufferer agony. It will have to be employed only for comfortable and dry damages or used as a secondary dressing to soak up exudates and shield the wound [28-29].

5.2. Hydrocolloid Dressing

Hydrocolloid dressings are amongst the most broadly used sauces. The term hydrocolloids describe the family of wound management products obtained from colloidal materials mixed with other substances equivalent to elastomers and adhesives. The everyday gel-forming marketers incorporate carboxymethylcellulose [CMC], gelatin, and pectin. Examples of hydrocolloid dressings include Granuflex, Tegasorb, etc. They occur in thin movies and sheets or as composite dressings that blend with other materials comparable to alginates. A randomized trial evaluating paraffin gauze and hydrocolloids dressings utilize to skin draft donor sites. The hydrocolloids achieve rapid medication and are much less painful dressings [30]. A difference is trained, involving patients with distress, a scratch produced by rubbing, and minor operations incisions, compared to a hydrocolloid dressing with non-adherent dressings. While time to heal used to be identical for both agencies, patients utilizing the hydrocolloids skilled much less ache, required less analgesia, and had been capable of carrying out their average everyday routine, including bathing or showering without affecting the dressing [31].

5.3. Alginate Dressings

The calcium and sodium salts of alginic acid and polysaccharide enclose the mannuronic acid and guluronic acid. Alginate dressings emerge either in the kind of stop dried permeable sheets or as bendy fibres, and the last showed for pressing pit wounds. Using alginates as dressings stems primarily from their ability to frame flex upon contact with wound exudates [32]. Alginates rich in man urinate, equivalent to sorbitan form gentle, flexible gels upon hydration. Those rich in guluronic acid, like kaltostat, kind less available gels upon absorbing wound oozes out. Some incorporate calcium alginate fibre reminiscent of sorbitan and tagged. When applied to wounds, ion gift within the alginate fibre is exchanged with these exudate and blood gifts to form a protecting film of gels. The gels help preserve the injurious unchanged in an organ's action at the choicest temperature, moisture content, and treatment temperature. The alginates' gelling property is to impute calcium ions, helping to cross-linked polymeric gels that degrade slowly. The capacity of calcium ions to forms crosslinks with the alginic acid polymer makes calcium alginate dressings ideal materials as scaffolds for tissue engineering [33].

5.4. Hydrogel Dressings

They are insoluble, hydrophilic substances produced using manufactured polymers, for example, polymethacrylates and polyvinyl pyrrolidine. Some dressings like Nu-gel and prison are alginate mix. It may be utilized both as an amorphous gel or elastic, solid sheet or films. The polymeric components are crosslinked so that they bodily entrap water. The sheets can soak up and maintain huge volumes of water upon contact to form and generate pus [34].

5.5. Semi-Permeable Adhesive Film Dressings

Film dressing was first made from nylon derivatives supporters in a sticky polyethene body, making them recondite. The standard nylon derived film dressing, nevertheless, have limited capability to soak up. Results within the accumulation of different exudates beneath bandages [35]. This leads to dermis maceration and bacterial proliferation, and the chance of illness. Accordingly, it requires ordinary altering as reasonable as irrigation of the wound with saline, making them unsuitable as wound dressings. The films can also be prominent, conform to contours such as elbows, knees, and sacral areas, and do not require further tapping. Nevertheless, they're skinny to be packed into deep or cavity wounds and handiest compatible with slightly shallow wounds [36].

5.6. Foam Dressings

It consists of porous polyurethane foam or films, generally with adhesive borders. Some foam dressings such as title have further wound contact layers to preclude adherence when the wound is dry. An occlusive polymeric backing layer restricts extra fluid loss and bacterial contamination [37]. Foam dressings hold a moist environment across the scars, provide thermal insulation, and are comfortable to wear. They're incredibly absorbent, absorbency being managed with foam properties such as texture, thickness, and pore measurement. The open-pore structure additionally vapours transmission price.

Froth dressings are not appropriate for dry epithelialiazing wounds or dehydrated scars as they rely upon dislike the polymer films to acquire a most productive injury recuperating condition. The sheets dressings shouldn't bc compatible as packs for cavity wounds though they may be used as a secondary dressing for wounds.

6. Wound Infections

The most widely recognized preventable test to wound recuperating is possible contagion, and topical antimicrobials have for quite some time been utilized observationally to attempt to anticipate wound disease. While microscopic organisms are a specific piece of the skin vegetation and wounds, a fundamental limit of 105 microbes has been proposed to depict colonization and clinically pertinent contamination that may block wound recuperating. It is additionally essential to recognize a coincidental positive culture and a genuine pathogen influencing an injury. Rehash surface societies in a wound are of restricted utilize, neither affirming nor discounting a proceeded with the disease; instead, clinical determination of a contaminated injury stays of essential significance. Profound tissue societies are, to some degree, more questionable. While they have better affectability and specificity in secluding a causative living being in a tainted injury, it is as yet not flawless; separates from various parts of a similar injury have even been appeared to have changed life forms. Generally, the specialist is intensifying the underlying damage with a considerably more profound injury; however, this may even now be an advantageous exchange off if it ensures suitable antimicrobial scope.

There are numerous methodologies for both treatment and anticipation of wound contaminations. Silver has been utilized as an assistant in twisted tend for more than 2000 years [68] and remains a well-known injury mind fixing today. It has an expansive range of movement and is accessible in various structures. More current advances in utilizing silver for wound recuperating have concentrated on considering the maintained arrival of silver in sufficiently high focuses to assess held adequacy. Nanocrystalline silver dressings were produced and help address the deficiency that silver nitrate has—to work legitimately, it would need to be managed 12 times each day.

Moreover, a current survey found no persuading proof that silver sulfadiazine has any impact on wound mending in general, notwithstanding its necessary use among specialists. Likewise, iodine-containing mixes have for some time been utilized as a part of wound mending; however, there have been a few worries with the danger of iodine-containing combinations, notably finished substantial injury territories. Yet, for constrained injuries, cadexomer (iodine inside a starch grid-shaped into microbeads) has a decent arrangement of information supporting its utilization as a suitable adjuvant for wound recuperating [38].

Various topical plans of anti-infection agents have additionally been produced. The rising confirmation has demonstrated the advantage of a discount on anti-infection balms. The genuine sign for topical antimicrobial is a clinically tainted injury—for example, purulent seepage, erythematic, warmth, agony, delicacy, or indurations. Various late investigations have reverberated this assessment. The routine anti-toxin treatment routine prompting no better results; however, it frequently brings about patient distress, alongside the likelihood of anti-toxin protection and contact dermatitis. The contact dermatitis is in a struggle with a couple of prior examinations where youngsters with minor scratches and creepy crawly chomps had lessened disease rates with topical antimicrobial salve, even though this can't be unmistakably summed up to all patients. Indeed, even after Moths micrographic surgery, a planned report found the rate of contamination after the clean surgical method to be under 1%, with the most astounding rate of diseases in fold terminations. According to all dermatology, utilization of topical anti-toxins ought to be held for conditions such as impetigo or an unmistakably contaminated injury [39].

7. Treatment Influences

The impacts of the entire scope of treatments cannot be considered in any considerable detail here. Still, preferably on a fundamental level, a treatment that is advantageous to the repair occasions is a treatment that fortifies instead of 'changes' the standard arrangement. Advancing or invigorating the incendiary circumstances isn't expected to accomplish a 'greater' inflammatory reaction, yet to amplify its effectiveness. Similarly, if delivering therapy during the proliferation phase, there would be no benefit in simply creating a more significant scar tissue volume. The advantage of appropriate intervention is that it stimulates a maximally efficient response, and therefore the required repair material is generated with the best quality and minimal time. In the renovating stage, the refinement of the scar tissue is the point. The utilization of treatment can have a substantial impact, particularly given the developing assortment of proof relating to the effects of mechanical pressure and collagen conduct [40].

References

[1] Lazaurus, G. S. Definitions and guidelines for the assessment of wounds and evaluation of heal ing, *Arch Dermatol.* 130.4 (1994) 489-493.

[2] Alonso, J. E. The management of complex orthopedic injuries, *Surg. Clin. N. America.* 76 (1996) 879-903.

[3] Robson, M. C., L. S. David and G. F. Michael, Wound healing: biologic features and approaches to maximize healing trajectories, *Curr. Problems surg.* 38 (2) (2001):72-140.

[4] Flangen, M. *The physiology of wound healing*, wound care 9 (2009) 299-300.

[5] Richardson, M. Acute wounds: an overview of the physiological healing process, *Nursing times* 100(4) (2004) 50-53.

[6] Komarcević, A. The modern approach to wound treatment, *Medicinski pregled* 53(7) (2000) 363-368.

[7] Percival, N. J. Classification of wounds and their management, *Surg.* 20(5) (2002) 114-117.

[8] Naradzay F. X. and R. Alson, *Burns thermal*, Web MD (2005).

[9] Harding, K. G., H. L. Morris and G. K. Patel, Clinical review Healing chronic wounds, *Br. Med. J.* 324 (2002) 160-163.

[10] Moore, K., R. McCallion, R,J. Searle, M.C. Stacey, K.G.Harding, Prediction and monitoring the therapeutic response of chronic dermal wounds, *INT Wound J.* 3(2006)89-96.

[11] Bolton, L. Wound dressings: meeting clinical and biological needs, *Dermatol. Nursing* 3(3) (1991)146-161.

[12] Kranser, D., K. L. Kennedy, B. S. Rolstad, A. W. Roma, The ABCs of wound care dressings, *Wound Manag.* 39(8) 68-69.

[13] Rothe, M. and V. Falanga, Growth factors: their biology and promise in dermatologic diseases and tissue repair, *Arch. Dermatol.* 125(10) (1989) 1390-1398.

[14] Shakespeare, P. Burn wound healing and skin substitutes, *Burns* 27(5) (2001) 517-522.

[15] Majumdar A. and P Sangole, Alternative Approaches to Wound Healing, Wound Healing: New Ins. *Anc. Chall.* (2016) 459.

[16] Glat P. M. and M. T. Longaker, *Wound healing Grabb and Smith's Plastic Surgery* 5th edn ed RW Beasley, CH Thorne and SJ Aston, (1997) 3-12.

[17] Greaves, N. S., K. J. Ashcroft, M. Baguneid and A. Bayat, Current understanding of molecular and cellular mechanisms in fibroplasia and angiogenesis during acute wound healing, *J. Derma. Sci.* 72(3) (2013) 206-217.

[18] Martin, P. Paul, Wound Healing--aiming for perfect skin regeneration, *Science* 276(5) (1997) 75-81.

[19] Bauer, S. M. Angiogenesis, vasculogenesis and induction of Healing in chronic wounds, *Vasc. Endovasc. Surg.* 39 (2005) 293-306.

[20] Miller, S. J., E. M. Burke, M.D. Rader, P.A. R.M. Lavker, Re-epithelialization of porcine skin by the sweat apparatus, *J. Inv. Dermatol.* 110(1)(1998) 13-19.

[21] Roh, C., S. Lyle, Cutaneous stem cells and wound healing, *Pedia. Res.* 59(S4) (2006), 100R.

[22] Werner, S., R. Grose, Regulation of wound healing by growth factors and cytokines, *Physiol. Rev.* 83 (2003)835-870.

[23] Jacinto, A., A. Martinez-Arias, P. Martin, Mechanisms of epithelial fusion and repair, *Nat. Cell Biology*. 3(5) (2001) 117.

[24] Tziotzios, C., C. Profyris, J. Sterling, Cutaneous scarring: Pathophysiology, molecular mechanisms, and scar reduction therapeutics: Part II. Strategies to reduce scar formation after dermatologic procedures, *J. Amer. Acad. Dermatol.* 66(1) (2012) 13-24.

[25] Profyris, C., Tziotzios, C. and Do Vale, I., 2012. Cutaneous scarring: Pathophysiology, molecular mechanisms, and scar reduction therapeutics: Part I. The molecular basis of scar formation, *J. Amer. Acad. Dermatol.* 66(1) (2012)1-10.

[26] Wollina, U., M. Kinscher, H. Fengler, Maggot therapy in the treatment of wounds of exposed knee prostheses, *Inter. J. Dermatol.* 44(10) (2005).884-886.

[27] Nigam, Y., A. Bexfield, S. Thomas, N. A. Ratcliffe, Maggot therapy: the science and implication for CAM part II—maggots combat infection, *Evidence-Based Compl. Alter. Med.* 3(3) (2006) 303-308.

[28] Khundkar, R., C. Malic, T. Burge, Use of Acticoat™ dressings in burns: what is the evidence, *Burns*, 36(6) (2010)751-758.

[29] Argenta, L. C., M. J. Morykwas, M. W. Marks, A. J. DeFranzo, J. A. Molnar, L. R. David, Vaccum –assissted closure: state of clinical art, *Plast. Reconstr. Surg.* 117 (7) (2006) 127-142.

[30] Quah, H. M., A. Maw, T. Young, D. J. Hay, Vaccum-assisted closure in the management of the open abdomen: a report of a case and initial experiences, *J. Tissue Viab.* 14 (2) (2004) 59-62.

[31] M. Kalpan, *Managing the open abdomen*, ostomy/wound Manag. 50(1) (2004) 2-8.

[32] Morin, R. J., Tomaselli, N. L. Interactive dressings and topical agents, *Clin. Plast. Surg.* 34(4) (2007)643-658.

[33] Dinah, F., A. Adhikari, Guaze packing of open surgical wounds: Empirical or evidence –based practice, *Ann. R. Coll. Surg. Engl.* 88 (2006) 33-36.

[34] Janis, J. E., R. K. Kwon, D. H. Lalonde, A practical guide to wound Healing, *Plast. Reconstr. Surg.* 125(6) (2010), 230-244.

[35] Jangde, R., D. Singh, Preparation and optimization of quercetin-loaded liposomes for wound healing, using response surface methodology, *Artif. Cells, Nanomed. Biotechnol.* (2014) 1-7.

[36] Wang, L., R. M. Shelton, P. R. Cooper, M. Lawson, J. T. Triffitt, J. E. Barralet, Evaluation of sodium alginate for bone marrow cell tissue engineering, *Biomat.* 24(20) (2003) 3475-3481.

[37] Boateng, J. S., K. H. Matthews, H. N. Stevens, G. M. Eccleston, Wound healing dressings and drug delivery systems: a review, *J. Pharm. Sci.* 97(8) (2008) 2892-2923.

[38] Ramos-e-Silva, M., D. C. M. Ribeiro, New dressings, including tissue-engineered living skin. *Clinic. Dermatol.* 20(6) (2002)715.

[39] Hansen, S. L., D. W. Voigt, P. Wiebelhaus, C. N. Paul, Using skin replacement products to treat burns and wounds, *Adv. Skin Wound Care*, 14(1) (2001) 37–45.

[40] Pham, C., J. Greenwood, H. Cleland, P. Woodruff, G. Maddern, Bioengineered skin substitutes for the management of burns: a systematic review, *Burns* 33(8) (2007) 946–957.

Chapter 2

ROLE OF THE PLANT IN WOUND HEALING

1. ROLE OF PLANTS IN WOUND HEALING

The wound is damage and injured tissue or the integral body's soft skin—the impairment due to the function and structure. Various plants are using many years ago to treat and care for wound healing and skin disorder in India's ancient times in rural and tribal places. Plants and plant products, active phytochemical constituents are found on plants. These are used in the treatment of healing of wounds and burns. These phytochemical constituents include various chemical families like alkaloids, essential oils, flavonoids, tannins, terpenoids, saponins, and phenolic compounds. Herbal extracts and plant products, and phytochemical actives parts have been of great interest to scientists to discover new effective drugs. (Ibukun, 2007) so many reports of antibacterials, anti-inflammatory activities have been studied vastly. Various data on pharmacology for plants and plant products are accepted throughout the world [1]. Bioactive compounds are phytochemicals present in food that help adjust metabolic processes and promote humans and animals' better health. The bioactive compound includes carotenoids, essential oil, antioxidants, or flavours widely incorporated into food products. These products are enhancing their sensory properties to develop their nutritional and health properties. The word “Bioactive” is composed of two words,” Bio and active.” Bios (in Greek ßio) refer to life, and Active (in Latin) means dynamic, full of energy, with energy or involve an activity. Bioactive compounds are a food component that influences physiological or cellular actions in the animal or human that consumes them [2].

1.1. Pharmacological Activity of Plant and Active Constituents for Wound Healing and Their Mechanism

1.1.1. VEGF and TGF- β mechanism

Wound activation of VEGF and TGF- β, activation of NF-B, activation of interleukin-8, increased expression ofiNOS and alpha-1 type-1 collagen, and anti-oxidant activity. Such as the hibiscus rosa Sinensis family of plants inducing the expression of VEGF and TGF- β. VEGF is responsible for angiogenesis. The factors are active on their respective receptors present in keratinocytes and macrophages, and they were inducing the essential functions during wound healing. Insufficient vascularization is a common feature of chronic and non-healing wounds. In animals (diabetic) have been researched for delayed wound healing. TGF- β acts on through the intracellular SMAD pathway, which regulates cell proliferation. TGF- β causes intracellular migration of leukocytes into the injured tissue. The factor of cell up-regulation in monocytes transform into macrophages. The area of debris and itself to release TGF- β and other growth factors, which in turn help in the formation of granulation tissue Activation of NF-B increases the pro-inflammatory which organizes and sustain the inflammatory processes which cause tissue damage; however, there are many reports are there that inhibition of NF-B may cause harmful effect to the organisms and sometimes it may cause inflammatory disease also. NF-B signalling has a significant role in maintaining the immune homeostasis in the epithelium cells. It is evaluated that the extract from herbs is used in the better wound healing process. The n-hexane extract of C. Officinalis has been examined to raise the activity of transcription factor NF-B in man immortalized keratinocytes and dermal fibroblast cells Interleukin-8 is a pro-inflammatory cytokine mechanism. Keratinocytes are rich in interleukin-8. The effect of interleukin-8 on migration and adhesion of HaCaT keratinocytes has been demonstrated. Its inhibits of phospholipase C (PLC-) is completely eradicated the migration of HaCaT keratinocytes. It is direct migration through the PLC pathway. Such as medicinal plant extracts and constituents activate the mechanism of interleukin-8. (e.g., the n-hexane extract C.officinalis is used to raise the activity of interleukin-8 in man's keratinocytes) [3].

The mechanism of nitric oxide is a small radical. The radical is the formation in the proprietary phase formation and increased iNOS expression release. The function of NO is in collagen generation proliferation and contraction of the cell. A high level of Polysaccharide extract is in C. ferrea is to rise the infection of iNOS. Alpha-1type-1 collagen encoded by Col 1 (I) gene. This gene participates in wound healing by producing the pro-alpha-1 (I) chain, type1 collagen. This pro-alpha-1 (I) chain is joined with the pro-alpha-1 (I) chain and with the pro-alpha-2 (I) chain to form pro-collagen, which undergo processing and rearrangement to produce type-1 collagen fibres. Rho family GTPase as Rac-1, Rho-A, and Cdc-42 plays a pivotal role in fibroblast cell proliferation and migration. Cell cycle regulators such as cyclins and cyclin-dependent kinase 1 and 2 are involved in cytoskeleton formation in fibroblasts. Many shreds of evidence suggest that wound experience oxidative stress due to a rise in neutrophils and MOP activity. This case causes the dissociation of a chronic wound. Production of reactive oxygen species (ROS) domino effect in cell toxicity via oxidative stress in chronic injury and delay wound healing.

Anti-oxidant activity of medicinal plants is due to the occurrence of various phytochemicals Naringenin the vital flavonoid, principally present in fruits; Citrus species and tomatoes and figs belong to Smyrna-type Ficuscarica. Naringetol; Salipurol; 4', 5, 7 Trihydroxy flavanone. Beneficial effects on the human body, such as adding metabolizing and acting as an antioxidant, anti-inflammatory, antibacterial. Hesperidin is flavanone glycosides occur in citrus fruits. Its aglycone form is hesperetin. It is consequent from "hesperidium," for fruit formed by citrus trees, such as orange, lemon, and food, peppermint. Hesperidin, collectively with other related bioflavonoids, was previously known as "vitamin P." Effect of hesperidin and insulin treatment on VEGF-c, Ang-1, Tie-2, TGF- β and Smad 2/3 mRNA expression in wound skin tissue of diabetic rats [4].

1.2. Myeloperoxidase

Many shreds of evidence suggest that the wound experience oxidative stress due to increased activity of neutrophils resultant oxidants and MPO activity. Increased activity of neutrophils resultant oxidants and MPO activity causes tissue damage in the chronic wound. Generation of reactive oxygen species (ROS) results in cell toxicity via oxidative stress in chronic wounds and delays wound healing. The antioxidant activity of medicinal plants is due to the presence of various phytochemicals [5].

1.2.1. Phytoconstituents of Herbal Plants Using in Wound Healing

1.2.1.1. Naringenin

Naringenin is one of the most important naturally-occurring flavonoids, predominantly found in some edible fruits, like Citrus species and tomatoes and figs belonging to Smyrna-type Ficuscarica. Other names: Naringetol; Salipurol; 4',5,7 Trihydroxyflavanone.

Beneficial effects on the human body, such as adding metabolizing and acting as an antioxidant, anti-inflammatory, antibacterial [6].

1.2.1.2. Hesperidin

Hesperidin is a flavanone glycoside found in citrus fruits. Its aglycone form is called hesperetin. Its name is derived from the word "hesperidium," for fruit produced by citrus trees, such as orange, lemon, and food, peppermint. It is a low molecular weight molecule (molecular weight 610.57 Da), with the bruto formula C28H34O15, and belongs to the flavanone class of flavonoids. IUPAC name: (2S)-5-hydroxy-2-(3-hydroxy-4-methoxyphenyl)-7- [(2S,3R,4S,5S,6R)-3,4,5-trihydroxy-6-[[(2R,3R,4R,5R,6S)- 3,4,5-trihydroxy-6-methyloxan-2-yl]oxymethyl]oxan-2- yl]oxy-2,3-dihydrochromen-4-one.Hesperidin, together with other similar bioflavonoids, was formerly called "vitamin P." Effect of hesperidin and insulin treatment on VEGF-c, Ang-1, Tie-2, TGF-β, and Smad 2/3 mRNA expression in wound skin tissue of diabetic rats [7].

1.2.1.3. Alkaloids

Alkaloids are physically involved, and heterocyclic compounds containing nitrogen atom in a ring system and side-chain imitation compounds of similar arrangement are also termed alkaloids. Alkaloids are also produced in dicot plants and lower plants monocots plants but in rare in monocot plants. Such alkaloids are not the first choice for wound healing, but they are indirectly used in wound healing. Essential oils are intense hydrophobic liquid that contains volatile compounds derived from plants. Generally, essential oils are extracted by distillation (e.g., by steam) essentials oils are used in the Healing of the wound, such as Lavender oil, chamomile oil, tea tree oil and thyme oil, Ocimum oil (basil), etc. [8].

1.2.2. Medicinal Plants Using in Wound Healing

1.2.2.1. Ghritkumari

Chemical constituents of aloe vera in haveanthraquinone derivative (10% to 40%); aloin, mucilage (30%), resinous substance (16% to 63%); aloesin as well as aloes one, sugars (about 25%), polysaccharides; acemannan and beta mannan, fatty acids as well as cholesterol, campesterol, P-sitosterol, glycoproteins (aloctins A and B), lectins, a gibberellin-like substance, enzymes such as cyclo-oxygenase and bradykininase, together with other compounds such as salicylic acid, cinnamic acid, phenol, and amino acids. Mechanism of action anti-inflammatory, antioxidant, flavonoids, tannins, and wound healing use in the excision model of wound healing apply [9].

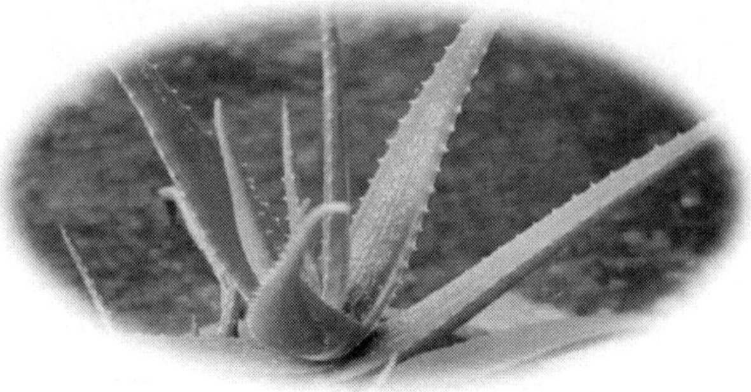

Figure 1. *Aloe vera* (Ghritkumari).

1.2.2.2. Pot Marigold

Chemical constituents are triterpenoids and flavonoids. No less than eight bioactive triterpenoid monoesters have been well-known in the extracts of dried calendula flowers: calenduladiol-3-O-palmitate and calenduladiol-3-O-myristate. The saponin fractions secluded from Calendula officinalis flower consist of oleanolic acid (205.53 mg/g dry weight) and ursolic acid. Mechanism of action Anti-oxidant, anti-inflammatory, wound healing. Generally uses in cutaneous wound healing and closure wound [10].

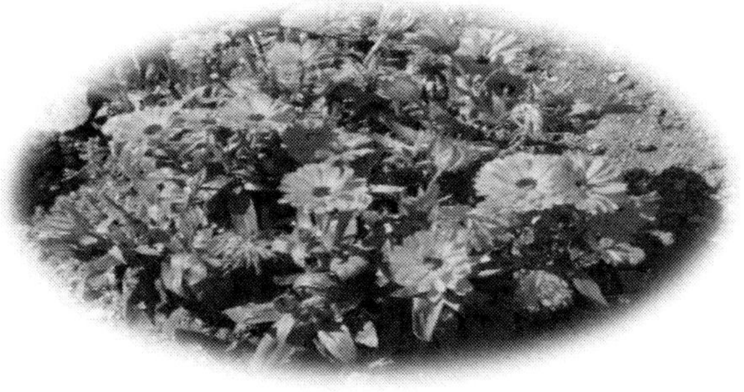

Figure 2. Marigold (Calendula officinalis).

1.2.2.3. Orange

Chemical constituents present in flavonoids. Steroids, hydroxy amides, alkanes, fatty acids, coumarins, peptides, carbohydrates, carbamates and alkylamines, carotenoids, volatile compounds, and nutritional elements, potassium, magnesium, calcium, and sodium. Mechanism of action Anti-oxidant, anti-inflammatory, cytokinin, wound Healing [11].

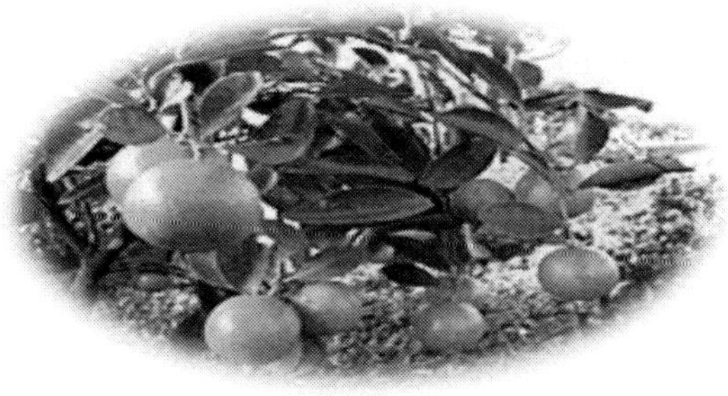

Figure 3. Orange (Citrus tamurana).

1.2.2.4. Turmeric

Chemical constituents presence in curcuminoids (3-6%), terpenoids, curcumin, glycosides, polysaccharides. Mechanism of action Anti-oxidant, anti-inflammatory, antibacterial, wound healing [12].

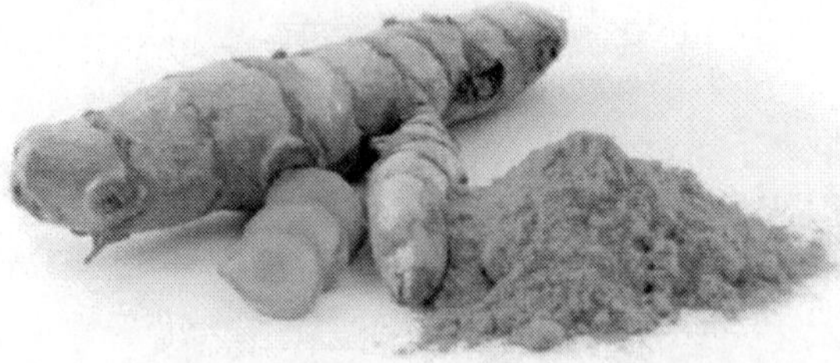

Figure 4. Turmeric (Curcuma longa).

1.2.2.5. Neem

Chemical constituents in presence triterpenoids, nimolicinol, nimocinol, azadirachtol, azadirachnol, nimbocinone, nimocinolide, isonimocinolide, nimocin and nimolinone, nonterpenoidal, components, nimbochalcin and nimbocetin. Mechanism of actionNimbidine, antioxidant, anti-inflammatory, antibacterial [13].

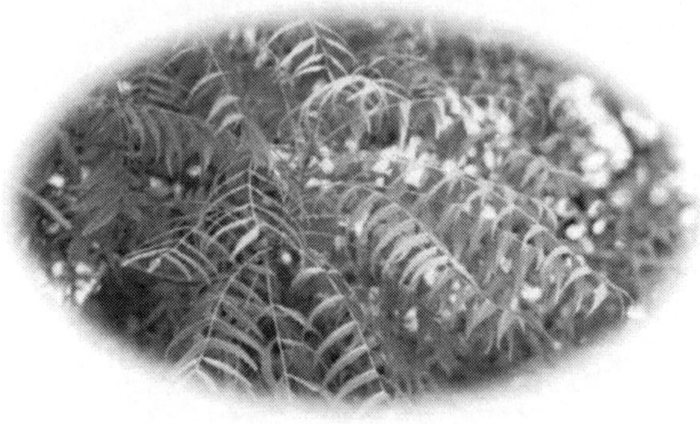

Figure 5. Neem (Azadirachtaindica).

1.2.2.6. Tulsi (Ocimum sanctum)

Chemical constituent presence in phenolic compounds, for example, curvilinear, circimaritin, isothymusin, apigenin and rosameric acid, and a considerable quantity of eugenol (Buddhadev, 2014). The leaves of Ocimum sanctum have 0.7% volatile oil comprised of 71% eugenol and

20% methyl eugenol. Mechanism of action Anti-inflammatory, antimicrobial, immune-stimulatory, flavonoids [14].

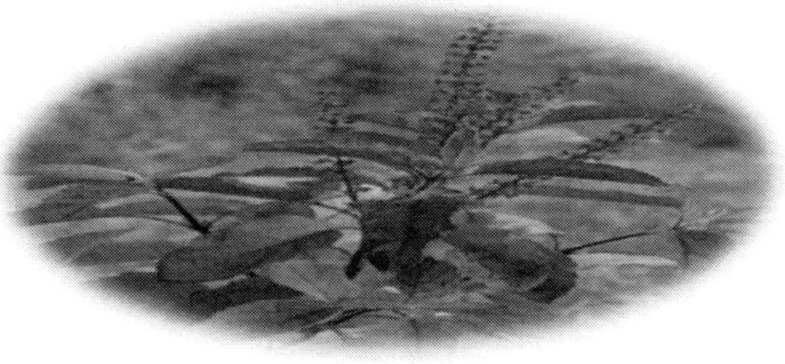

Figure 6. Tulsi (Ocimum sanctum).

1.2.2.7. Guildhall

Chemical constituent's presence β-sitosterol, stigmasterol, taraxeryl acetate, and three cyclopropane compounds and their derivatives. Flowers contain flavonoids and vitamins, thiamine, riboflavin, niacin, and ascorbic acid. Mechanism of action Anti-oxidant, anti-inflammatory, wound healing [15].

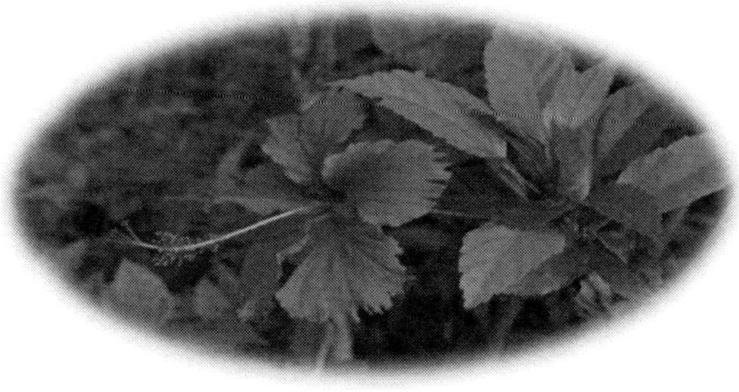

Figure 7. Gudhal (Hibiscus rosa-sinensis).

Table 1. Evidence based medicinal plants and parts used in wound healing

S. No.	Botanical name	Part used	Wound healing model used	Ref
1	Acoruscalamu	Green leaves	Excision and incision	[8]
2	Allium sativum	Bulb	Excision, incision and dead space	[7]
3	Adhatodavasica	Leaves	Excision	[6]
4	Alternantherabrasiliana	Leaves	Excision and incision	[9]
5	Andrographispaniculata	Whole plant	Excision	[9]
6	Areca catechu	Fruit	Burn wound	[10]
7	Buteamonosperma	Root,	Excision, incision and dead space	[11]
8	Cassia fistula	Fuits,stem	Incision	[12]
9	Catharanthusroseus	Leaves	Excision, incision and dead space	[13]
10	Carica papaya	Leaves	Excision, incision and dead space	[13]
11	Cordiadichotoma	Leaves	Burn wound	[14]
12	Desmodiumtriquetrum	Leaves	Excision, incision and dead space	[16]
13	Embeliaribes	Rhizomes	xcision, incision and dead space	[9]
14	Ficusreligiosa	Fruits,root	Excision, incision and dead space	[8]
15	Gentian lutea	Root,stem	Excision and incision	[9]
16	Glycyrrhizaglabra	Leaves, stem, and flower	Excision and	
17	Incision	[10]		
18	Gymnema Sylvestre	Leaves, stem, and flower	Excision and	
19	Incision	[13]		
20	Heliotropiumindicum	Whole plant	Excision	[12]
21	Indigoferaenneaphylla	Whole plant	Excision	[16]
22	asminumauriculatum	Juice of leaves	Incision	[14]
23	Kaempferia galangal	Rhizomes	Excision and incision	[17]

S. No.	Botanical name	Part used	Wound healing model used	Ref
24	Lycopodiumserratum	Whole plant	Excision	[16]
25	Mimosa pudica	Whole plant	Excision, incision, and dead space	[14]
26	Mimusopselengi	Leaves	Excision, incision, and dead space	[16]
27	Micheliachampaca	Stem,bark	Excision and burn wound	[11]
28	Mirabilis jalapa	Flower	Excision and incision	[10]
29	Piper betel	Tuberous root	Excision	[12]
30	Quercusinfectoria	Leaves and stem bark	Excision	[13]

REFERENCES

[1] A, G. P. (2013). Phytoextract in wound healing. *Journal of Pharmacy and Pharmaceutical Sciences*, 16:760-820.

[2] Abu-Al-Basal, M. (2001). *The influence of some local medicinal plant extracts on skin wound healing activity*. Evaluated by histological and ultra.

[3] AK, S. H. (2012). A recent update of botanicals for wound healing activity. *International Research Journal of Pharmacy*., 3:1-7.

[4] Akihisa, Y. (1996). 4. Akihisa T, Yasukawa K, Oinuma H, KasaharaTriterpene alcohol from the flowers of compositae and their anti-inflammatory effects. *Phytochemistry*, 43:1225-1260.

[5] Akkol, E. (2009). *Ethanopharmacol.* 124-137.

[6] Alonso J. E Lee J, B. A. (1996). The management of complex orthopaedic injuries. *The management of complex orthopaedicinjuries.*, 879-903.

[7] Bowler P. G., Duerden B. I., Armstrong D. G. Wound Microbiology and Associated Approaches to Wound Management. *Clin Microbiol Rev*. 2001 Apr; 14(2):244–69.

[8] Jain N, J. R. (2010). Evaluation of wound-healing activity of Acoruscalamus. *Natural Product Research*, 24:534-541.

[9] LotlekarResha, M. S. (2011). Screening of Allium sativum bulb for wound healing and antioxidant activities. *International Journal of Pharmaceutical Sciences*, 3:1292-1298.

[10] Sundar, K. G. (2010). Wound healing effect of various extracts of Adhatodavasica. *International Journal of Pharma and Bio Sciences.*, 1:530-536.

[11] Barua C. C., T. A. (2009). Wound healing activity of methanolic extract of leaves of Alternantherabrasiliana using in-vivo and in-vitro model. *Wound healing activity of Indian Journal of Experimental Biology* 2009, 47:1001-1005.

[12] Mohanty A, P. D. (2010). Mohanty A Preliminary pytochemical screening and wound healing activity of Andrographispeniculata. *Journal of Chemical and Pharmaceutical Research*, 2:649-654.

[13] Bharat M, V. D. (2014). Ethanolic extract of oral Areca catechu promotes burn wound healing in rats. *International Journal of Pharmaceutical Sciences Review and Research*, 25:145-148.

[14] Muralidhar A, B. K. (2011). Evaluation of wound healing properties of bioactive fractions from the extract of Buteamonosperma (Lam).stem bark. *International Journal of Phytomedicine,* 3:4149.

[15] Nurismail, E. (2003). *Antimicrobial and wound healing activities of three Cassia Master of Science*. Faculty of Medicine and Health Sciences. Universiti Putra Malaysia.

[16] Nayak B. S., P. L. (2006). *Catharanthusroseus flower extract has wound-healing activity in SpraguaDawley BMC Complementary and Alternative Medicine*, 6:1-6.

[17] NS, G. S. (2019). Wound healing properties of Carica papaya latex: in-vivo evaluation of mice burn model. *Journal of Ethanopharmacology*, 121:338-341.

Chapter 3

NOVEL CARRIER SYSTEM

1. INTRODUCTION

A novel carrier system is a novel approach to drug delivery that addresses conventional drug delivery systems' limitations. Recent medicine cures a scrupulous disease by targeting precisely the affected zone and transporting the drug to that area. The drug carrier system is administered to the patient. It reaches the specific 'site of action.' Some carrier systems and drug targeting systems are presently under development to minimize drug degradation and loss, prevent harmful side effects and increase drug bioavailability. The fraction of the drug accumulated in the required zone, Various drug carriers, is reported, such as soluble polymers, microparticles made of insoluble or biodegradable natural and synthetic polymers, microcapsules, cells, cell ghosts, lipoproteins, liposome's and micelles [1]. The carriers can be made sometimes targeted to the site (e.g., Conjugation of the airline with specific antibodies against definite characteristic components of the desirable site), slowly degradable, and stimuli-reactive (e.g., pH- or temperature-sensitive). Targeting is the capability to express the drug-loaded system to the desired location. For defining the selected sites for drug release, two effective mechanisms can be addressed: (i) passive and (ii) active targeting. Superior accumulation of chemotherapeutic agents in solid tumors is a better example of passive targeting due to the improved vascular permeability of tumor tissues compared with healthy tissue. Receptors accept drug carriers' actions with ligand to the desired cell's surface area is a well-known example of active targeting.

Developing a successful formulation for controlled drug release important parameter is biodegradation. Prospective release mechanisms involve (i) diffusion of surface-bound / adsorbed drugs; (ii) dispersion through the carrier surrounding substance; (iii) transmission through the carrier wall; (iv) matrix erosion of carrier system and (v) diffusion of combined of matrix carrier. By different administration modes of medicine, a drug's choice has frequently influenced the drug delivery system's success and failure [2]. Degradation and diffusion of polymer, the drug's release rate are controlled and sustained in the drug delivery system. Sometimes various compounds of herbal extracts will degrade in the highly acidic pH of the stomach. Before reaching the blood, few compounds might be metabolized by the liver, and due to this necessary quantity of the drug may not arrive in the blood. The drug will not show any therapeutic effect if the drug does not reach the blood at a minimum level known as 'minimum effective level.'Phytopharmaceuticals compounds are traditional medicine obtained from natural resources as an alternative to synthetic drugs. Natural constituents are more just and rapidly metabolized in the body. Phytomedicines have fewer side effects and enhance absorption in blood circulation, shows more effective treatment than the synthetic drug. Besides, if phytomedicines are single or purified, they can become easily standardized and used for novel drug delivery systems [3].

2. Novel Carrier Systems

2.1. Liposomes

Liposomes are the self-assembled closed structures having the size range of 0.05-5.0 μm in diameter, entrapping solvent in its interior core. Liposomes are admired for their unique property of amphiphilicity, having a lipophilic and hydrophilic group on the same molecules. Liposome membranes are composed of phospholipids that can be naturally-derived or obtained synthetically with defined acyl chains and head groups. The phospholipids align themselves in a manner having an orientation for both the lipophilic core and hydrophilic core. Thus the bi-orientation allows entrapment of both lipophilic and hydrophilic drugs, either in the phospholipids bilayer/ in the entrapped aqueous volume [4].

Liposome was first developed in England by Alec D in 1961. Bangham, who studied phospholipids and blood clotting, reported that phospholipids, when coming in contact with water, immediately form a sphere because one end of each molecule was water-soluble. In contrast, the opposite end is water-insoluble as its vesicular amphiphilic nature dragged inventors to use liposomes as efficient delivery systems. Topical drug delivery is an attractive route for local and systemic treatment. Liposomes are advantageous in terms they protect the drug from degradation, gives better absorption in the skin because it has an affinity to permeate through the skin, reduces the side effect of the drug by lowering the dose amount, and enhances the solubility of the poorly soluble drug. In the formulation of topical dosage forms, attempts are being made to utilize drug carriers that ensure adequate localization or penetration of drug within or through the skin to enhance the local and minimize the systemic effects or to provide acceptable percutaneous absorption[1] Liposomal formulations have been used to administer medications by several routes such as the oral, parenteral. Topical among all topical courses has been considered a promising way for helping drugs because of its accessibility and large surface. Due to their versatility and clinical efficacy, liposomes have been widely used to promote the dermal delivery of drugs that have to act topically and enhance transdermal delivery of drugs intended for systemic use exploiting non-invasive and alternative routes to oral administration [5].

2.2. Phyto-Vesicles

Molecular complexes developed by using lipid compatible with incorporating plant extracts /water-soluble constituents. Which significantly improves the bioavailability of bioactive components known as Phyto-vesicles pyrosomes. Phytosomes are manifested to enhance the poorly soluble drugs' solubility with increased bioavailability due to active absorption through the GIT. The differentiating factor between liposomes and Phyto-vesicles is in liposomes. The active components are dissolved in the medium contained in the cavity or the layers of the membranes.

In contrast, in the Phyto-vesicles, it is a whole part of the membrane, being the molecule affixed through chemical bonds to the phospholipids' polar head. It has determined the formation of hydrogen bonds between the polar heads of phospholipids (Phosphate and ammonium) and the substrate's polar functionalities spectroscopically. Secondly, the difference lies in the association of molecules that are in the photo-vesicle. A unit consists of as few as two molecules (one PC plus one polyphenol).

Table 1. Herbal formulations based on liposomal drug delivery system

Formulation	Active Ingredients	Application	Biological Activity	Ref
Ampelopsin liposomes	Ampelopsin	Improved outcomes	Anticancer	[5]
Atractylodes liposomes	Atractylodes macrocephaly	Enhancement of solubility and bioavailability	Digestive disorders and anti-cancer	[6]
Capsaicin liposomes	Capsaicin	Prolong action, permeation enhancement	Analgesic	[4]
Curcumin liposomes	Curcumin	Long systemic residence time and high entrapment efficiency	Anticancer	[11]
Garlicin liposomes	Garlicin	Enhanced therapeutic outcomes	Lungs	[13]
Magnolol liposomes	Magnolol	Efficacy enhancement	Vascular smooth muscle proliferation inhibition	[7]
Myrtus communis liposomes	Myrtus communis	Activity enhancement	Antimicrobial and anti oxidant	[10]
Nux vomica liposomes	strychin	Improved stability	Antineoplastic, anti inflammatory	[8]
Paclitaxel liposomes	Paclitaxel	Sensitivity towards pH and improved entrapment efficiency	Anticancer	[7]
Puerarin liposomes	Puerarin	Enhanced efficacy	Antioxidant and anti hypercholesterolemic	[6]
Quercetin liposomes	Quercetin	Improved bioavailability and side effect reduction	inflammatory and analgesic	[5]
Flavonoids liposomes	Quercetin and Rutin	Hemoglobin binding enhancement	Hemoglobin	[3]
Tripterygium wilfordi liposomes	Tripterygium wilfordi	Improved stability	Anticancer	[14]

Table 1. (Continued)

Formulation	Active Ingredients	Application	Biological Activity	Ref
Usnic acid liposomes	Usnic acid	Prolong action and solubility enhancement	Anti mycobacterial	[11]
Wogonin liposomes	Wogonin	Prolong duration of action	Anticancer	[10]
Silymarin	Silymarin	Improve bioavailability	Hepatoprotective	[9]
Artemisia arborescens essential oil	Artemisia	Targeting of essential oils to cells enhance penetration into, cytoplasmatic barrier	Antiviral	[8]
Colchicine	Colchicine	Enhance skin accumulation, prolong drug release and improve site-specific	Antigout	[10]
Catechins	Catechins	Increased permeation through skin	Antioxidant and chemopreventive	[6]
Diospyrin	Diospyrin	Enhancement of its anti-tumor effect	Anti-cancer activity	[3]
Myrtus communis	Myrtisin	Increase in its activities	Antioxidant and antimicrobial activity	[9]

Table 2. Herbal formulations based on phytosomes drug delivery system

Formulation	Active ingredients	Application	Ref
Silymarin phytosome	silymarin	increase in its oral bioavailability	[7]
IdB1016	silymarin	Improved bioavailability of silybin	[6]
Silymarin phytosome	silymarin	High inter-patient variability	[4]
Silipide phytosome	Silipide	Excellent tolerability	[7]
Silymarin phytosome	silymarin	increase in the duration of action	[6]
Siliphos[R]	silipide and silybin	Improved gastrointestinal absorption and oral bioavailability of IdB1016.	[4]
Silybin phytosome	silybin	A decrease in levels of hepatic enzymes ALT and AST	[5]
Grape seed phytosome	procyanidins	increase in the duration of action	[10]
Grape seed phytosome	procyanidins	elevated blood TRAP (Total Radical trapping Antioxidant	[11]
Leucoselectphytosome			[13]
Green select Phytosome	catechins	Improve Absorption of green tea	[14]
Herba Epimedii flavonoids phytosome	icariin	Enhanced oil/water apparent partition coefficient of icariin	[11]
Ginkgoselect phytosome	Ginkgo biloba	Absorption of ginkgolides A & B	[13]
Quercetin pytosome	quercetin	Improved therapeutic efficacy	[9]
Curcuminphospholipid complex	curcumin	Improved absorption	[7]
Naringenin phospholipid complex	Naringenin	longer duration of action	[6]
Ginkgo biloba phytosome	Ginkgo biloba	Increased its action	[8]
Curcumin phytosomes	Curcumin	Improved antioxidant activity and bioavailability	[9]
Embelin phytosomes	Embelin	Solubility enhancement	[8]
Epigallocatechin phytosomes	Epigallocatechins	Absorption enhancement	[12]
Ginkgo biloba phytosomes	Ginkgo biloba	Improved efficacy	[13]

Table 2. (Continued)

Formulation	Active ingredients	Application	Ref
Ginsenosides phytosomes	Ginsenosides	Absorption enhancement	[18]
Hawthorn phytosomes	Hawthorn	Improved efficacy and absorption	[10]
Marsupium phytosomes	Marsupium	Bioavailability enhancement	[6]
Naringenin phytosomes	Naringenin	Prolong action and enhanced bioavailability	[15]
Oxymatrine phytosomes	Oxymatrine	Bioavailability enhancement	[20]
Procyanidins phytosomes	Procyanidins	Increased total radical trapping antioxidant parameter (TRAP)	[14]

In contrast, a liposome unit is an aggregate of hundreds of phospholipids molecules into a spherule, within which other molecules are compartmentalized but not specifically bonded. Thirdly in terms of oral delivery, Phyto vesicles are more than liposomes [6]. Various Phyto-vesicles herbal formulations are given in Table 2. Phyto-vesicles' membrane nature allowed easy permeation through the non-lipophilic membrane and absorbed better in the intestinal lumen. Even small Phyto vesicles' small measures could be highly effective due to appreciating bioavailability and assure delivery, which will have high clinical benefits [7].

2.3. Microspheres

Microspheres are matrix particles of size range1-300 μm. These matrix particles can be fabricated using various polymers with biodegradable or non-biodegradable characteristics such as polyethylene, polydextran, albumin, Gelatin, Modified Starch, Polypropylene, Dextran, Polylactic acid. The drug release profile of microspheres could be altered by modifying the polymer matrix's disintegration and dissolution behavior. Alteration can be accomplished by adjusting size, structure, polymer concentration, or co-introduction of additional polymers. These matrix systems are not only used for the incorporation of synthetic drugs. Still, they could also incorporate active plant ingredients, such as extract of rutin, camptothecin, zedoary oil, tetrandrine, quercetin, and Cynara scolymus has been made into microspheres for wound healing (Table 6). The actives' sustained release with enhanced bioavailability is achieved by formulating camptothecin extract with anti-inflammatory activity into microspheres for prolonged release of the drug (12 hours). Similarly, the micro matrix prepared by emulsion-solvent diffusion method of Zedoary turmeric oil into microspheres supported sustained release [8].

Table 3. Herbal formulations based on microsphere drug delivery system

Formulation		Application	Biological Activity	Ref
Camptothecin Microsphere	Camptothecin	Dose reduction	Anticancer	[8]
Ginsenosides Microsphere	Ginsenosides	Solubility and stability improvement	Anticancer	[10]
Piper sarmentosumn Microsphere	Piper sarmentosumn	Easy for industrial scale-up	Antidiabetic	[7]
Quercetin Microsphere	Quercetin	Permeation enhanced	Anti-inflammatory and antioxidant	[12]
Rutin Microsphere	Rutin	Specific delivery to heart and brain vascular systems	Anti oxidant	[13]
Silymarin Microsphere	Silymarin	Sustained release of medicament Improved patient compliance	Treatment of Liver diseases	[8]

2.4. Nanoparticles

The nanoparticle is a collective name for nanospheres and nanocapsules. Nanospheres have a matrix type structure, and nanoparticles surface are entrapped or dissolved in the matrix active compounds can be adsorbed. Nanocapsules have a polymeric shell and an inner core. The active substances are usually dissolved in the middle and adsorbed at their surface in the inner core. Nanoparticles or colloidal carriers have been extensively investigated in biomedical and biotechnological areas, especially in drug delivery systems for drug targeting. Their particle size (ranging from 10 to 1000 nm) is acceptable for intravenous injection. Depending on the desired administration way, the size of the carriers should be optimized. Thus, if the carrier size is under 1 m, an intravenous injection (the diameter of the smallest blood capillaries is 4 m) is enabled, and this carrier size is also desirable for intramuscular and subcutaneous administration, minimizing any possible irritant reactions [9].

2.5. Nanoemulsions and Microemulsion

Nanoemulsions, a well-known name in the area of formulation because of its high potential in pharmaceutics, biotechnology, cosmaceuticals, and nutraceuticals, consists of deformable dispersed droplets in the range below 5 nm. It is an anisotropic combination of oils with surfactants and co-surfactants that form fine oil-in-water (O/W) or water-in-oil emulsions (W/O) with a droplet size usually below 500 nm. It requires external energy to break large droplets into a nano size. No spontaneous formation of droplets occurs; extreme shear is necessary to overcome surface tension's effects to rupture the droplets into thc nanoscale. It is also established that nanoemulsions require a lesser quantity of surfactant compared to microemulsions. These systems are highly acceptable because of the solubility enhancing property of poorly soluble drugs, high permeability due to surfactant, and wide distribution of drugs, which will increase bioavailability. The emulsion particle size will protect the drugs from hydrolyzation; thus, the herbal drug's nanoemulsions could prove beneficial in all terms. Many plant extracts are formulated into emulsions such as camptothecin, Brucea javanica oil, coixenolide oil, and zedoary oil [10].

2.6. Niosomes

The Substance, those are formed microscopic lamellar structures with subsequent hydration in an aqueous medium called niosomes. Niosomes are a mixture of cholesterol, non-ionic surfactant, and charge inducing agents.

Table 4. Herbal formulations based on nanoparticles drug delivery system

Formulation	Active Ingredients	Application	Biological Activity	Ref
Artemisinin nanoparticles	Artemisinin	Bioavailability enhancement and sustained drug delivery	Anticancer	[6]
Berberine nanoparticles	Berberine	Inhibition of Helicobacter pylori growth	Anticancer	[9]
Breviscapin nanoparticles	Breviscapin	Prolong half-life	Cerebrovascular and cardiovascular	[15]
Camptothecin nanoparticles	Camptothecin	Prolong circulation and high-density around tumor containing the area	Anticancer	[12]
Cuscuta Chinensis nanoparticles	Cuscuta Chinensis	Solubility enhancement	Antioxidant and liver protective	[13]
Ginkgo biloba nanoparticles	Ginkgo biloba	Metabolism and cerebral blood flow improvement	Brain activator	[8]
Ginseng nanoparticles	Ginseng	Improved Stability and pharmacological response	Anti oxidant	[10]
Glycyrrhizic acid nanoparticles	Glycyrrhizic acid	Bioavailability enhancement	Antihypertensive and anti-inflammatory	[11]
Hypocrellins nanoparticles	Hypocrellins	Improved efficacy, hydrophilicity, and stability	Antiviral	[18]
Paclitaxel nanoparticles	Paclitaxel	Sustained action and minimization of side effects	Anti cancer	[16]
Paclitaxel doxorubicin nanoparticles	Paclitaxel doxorubicin	Lesser chances of resistance development	Anti cancer	[17]
Quercetin nanoparticles	Quercetin	Improved therapeutic outcome and release enhancement	Anti oxidant	[15]

Formulation	Active Ingredients	Application	Biological Activity	Ref
Radix Salvia Miltiorrhiza nanoparticles	Radix Salvia Miltiorrhiza	Bioavailability enhancement	Anti anginal	[16]
Silibinin nanoparticles	Silibinin	Improved entrapment and stability	Hepatoprotective	[11]
Tetrandrine nanoparticles	Tetrandrine	Sustained release of drug	Lungs	[14]
Naringenin nanoparticles	Naringenin	Solubility enhancement and improved release of drug	Hepatoprotective	[12]
Zedoary turmeric oil nanoparticles	Zedoary turmeric oil	Improved stability and improved loading of drug	Liver protective, Anti oxidant and anti neoplastic	[13]
Hypocrellins	Hypocretin	Improved performance in both stability and hydrophilicity	Antiviral activity	[8]
Tripterygium wilfordii	Triptolide	Enhance the penetration of drugs through the stratum corneum by increased hydration	Anti-inflammatory	[20]
Flavonoids and lignans	Rutin	Improve water solubility	Hepatoprotective and antioxidant effects	[24]
Artemisia	Artemisinin	Sustained drug release	Anticancer Anti-inflammatory	[26]
paclitaxel	Taxel	Enhance the bioavailability and sustained drug release	Anticancer	[24]
silymarin	Silibinin	High entrapment efficiency and stability	Hepatoprotective	[20]
Curcuma long	Curcuminoids	Prolonged-release of the curcuminoids	Anticancer and antioxidant	[20]
Podophyllum emodi	Camptothecin	Prolonged blood circulation and high accumulation in tumors	Anticancer	[12]

Niosomes contains hydrophobic and hydrophilic layer and formed drug molecules having a wide range of solubility. Niosomes are assessed in various pharmaceutical applications. Niosomes, which are prepared by encapsulation of treatment agents, can minimize systemic toxicity and clearance of such agents from the body with slow drug release.

Modification in drug release rate can be achieved by changing in composition vesicles of niosomes for drug reservoirs, controlled release, permeation enhancement of drugs, and drug targeting. The potential of carrying various drug niosomes is used in a drug delivery system, both hydrophobic drugs (in lipid area) and hydrophilic drugs (by loading in inner space). Encapsulated niosomes have less systemic absorption of topical delivery that targets the skin's infected area in various diseases like skin cancer and wounds [11]. To improve multiple functions on different skin levels (skin surface, epidermis, dermis, and hypodermis), the topical drug delivery system is started. However, various limitations are reported in traditional topical preparations, e.g., less percutaneous diffusion because of the barrier function of the stratum corneum and absorption to the systemic circulation in the present scenario niosomes are a popular, topical drug delivery system because of having excellent characteristics such as improved diffusion of drugs, the capability to carry both hydrophilic and lipophilic drugs and significant, sustained drug release pattern [12].

2.7. Proniosomes

Proniosomes are the dry formulation of water-soluble carrier particles that are coated with a surfactant (use on agitation in hot aqueous media within minutes rehydration of proteasomes) [13].

Proniosomes, which is one of the nanotechnology advancements, minimize problems of vesicular systems such as aggregation, fusion, and leakage of drug and provide additional convenience in transportation, distribution, storage, and dosing [14]. It improves the oral bioavailability, targets drugs to the specific site, and infiltrates drugs across the stratum corneum. It lengthens the survival of the drug in systemic circulation and finally minimizes the toxicity.

2.8. Ethosomes

Ethosomes are lipid vesicles composed of phospholipids and a high concentration of ethanol and water. They can form multilamellar vesicles and entrapment capability for various lipophilicities molecules; however, they differ from liposomes in composition (high content of ethanol). Compared to traditional liposomes, ethosomes show smaller vesicle size, superior entrapment competence, and enhanced stability [15]. To provide sustained delivery of drugs, those formulations act as reservoir systems. Ethosomes may be unilamellar or multilamellar through to the core when visualizing by transmission electron microscopy [16]. Using various methods of preparation, composition, and application of techniques like sonication, ethosomes vesicle size can be achieved from tens of nanometre to a few microns. For a better drug delivery system in occlusive and non-occlusive conditions ethosomes play an essential role [17]. The elastic vesicles and transferases have also been used as drug carriers for a range of small molecules, peptides, proteins, and vaccines. For better penetration power to deeper skin and blood circulation layers, ethosomes enhance the carrier system in drug delivery. Ethosomes are formulated by hot and cold methods for both lipophilic and hydrophilic drugs, e.g., Ammonium glycyrrhizinate ethosomal suspension (Table 5) prepared for the topical application and treatment of the inflammatory diseases of the skin [18]. Enhance permeability and bioavailability of the drug found to be safe when applied for 24 hours of topical administration in the form of ethosomes suspension. Triptolide ethosomes formulated for topical delivery of the Triptolide shows an enhanced bioavailability due to an increase in the accumulation and reduction in erythema more speedily than the other formulations [19].

Table 5. Herbal formulations based on emulsion systems

Formulation		Application	Biological Activity	Ref
Azadirachta Indica emulsion	Azadirachtin	Reduction in associated adverse reactions	Acaricidal, anti bacterial and anti fungal	[13]
Berberine emulsion	Berberine	More residence time in the body	Anticancer	[14]
Curcumin emulsion	Curcumin	Improved absorption	Anticancer	[20]
Docetaxel emulsion	Docetaxel	More residence time in the body	Anticancer	[21]
Matrine emulsion	Matrine	Sustained release of medicament	Anti-inflammatory and anti bacterial	[22]
Quercetin emulsion	Quercetin	Permeability enhancement	Anti oxidant	[8]
Rhubarb emulsion	Rhubarb	Therapy improvement	Laxative and cathartic	[12]
Zedoary turmeric Oil emulsion	Zedoary turmeric oil	Dispersibility, stability and bioavailability enhancement	Liver protective, anti-cancer and anti Bacterial	[11]

Table 6. Herbal formulations based on transferosomal drug delivery systems

Formulation		Application	Biological activity	References
Colchicine transferases	Colchicine	Reduction in associated GIT side effects	Antigout	[18]
Curcumin transferases	Curcumin	Permeation enhancement	Anticancer and anti oxidant	[19]

2.9. Transfereosomes

Transferosomes are potential drug delivery for the topical administration of the drug as phospholipid vesicles can easily penetrate through the skin and overcome the difficulty of penetration throughout the stratum corneum [20].

Transferosomes have physicochemical properties of drugs immeasurably contributed to overcoming problems faced by topical drug administration drug delivery such as incapable of penetration through the stratum corneum, transporting larger molecules, and the rate-limiting step their transport through the skin in the development of novel approaches [21]. Transfersomes improve penetration power in the stratum corneum, consequences from hydration or osmotic force in the skin's skin intracellular pores due to their flexibility. That can respond to external pressure by rapid and energetically inexpensive shape transformations of optimized particles or vesicles. These elastic vesicles can constrict themselves transport larger molecules through skin pores, many times smaller than their size. Both formulation Transferosomes and Ethosomes are coated with phospholipid vesicles and drug administration via transdermal route and improving the stratum corneum barrier's penetration power. Still, its action of different transferases has to utilize the osmotic pressure and hydration of the skin. In the case of ethosomes, it has enhanced the drug's solubility because they have a high ethanol content (20-45%). Ethanol is a chemical permeation enhancer. It disrupts the membrane barrier [22] in the novel carrier systems used herbal constituents in the upper layers of skin while for deeper layer and systemic delivery [23].

References

[1] Khemariya, P., Jain, A., Goswami, R., Bhargava, & Singhal, S. K. (2010). Advances in Novel Drug Delivery Carriers: Formulation

and *In Vitro* Evaluation of Solid Lipid Nanoparticles of Nateglinide. *International Journal of Pharmaceutical and Applied Sciences*, 1(1), 104-108.

[2] Biju, S. S., Talegaonkar, S., Mishra, P. R., & Khar, R. K. (2006). Vesicular system: an overview. *Indian J Pharm*, 68(2), 141-153.

[3] Atmakuri, L. R., & Dathi, S. (2010). Current trends in herbal medicines. *J Pharm Res*. 3(1),109-113.

[4] Sinico, C., Logu, A. D., & Lai, F. (2005). Liposomal incorporation of *Artemisia arborescens* L. essential oil and *in vitro* antiviral activity. *Eur J Pharm Biopharm*, 59(1),161-168.

[5] Straubinger, R. M., & Balasubramanian, S. V. (2005). Preparation and characterization of Taxane containing liposomes. *Methods Enzymol*. 39(1), 97-117.

[6] Bisht, S., Feldmann, G., & Soni, S. (2007). Polymeric nanoparticle encapsulated curcumin: a novel strategy for human cancer therapy. *J Nanobiotech,* 5(3).101-105.

[7] Mei, Z., Chen, H., Weng, T., Yang, Y., & Yang, X. (2003). Solid lipid nanoparticle and microemulsion for topical delivery of triptolide. *Eur J Pharm Biopharm*, 56,189-196.

[8] Chauhan, N. S., Rajan, G., & Gopalakrishna, B. (2009). A potential phytophospholipid carrier for herbal drug delivery. *J Pharm Res,* 2(7),1267-1270.

[9] Dubey, D., Shrivastva, S., Gangwal, A., & Dubey, P. K. (2010). *Phytosomes: A Novel Dosage structure*. URL: http://www. Pharmainfo.net.

[10] Kannaiyan, S., Muthuprasanna, P. & Vardhareddy, V. (2009). Effect of carbopol gel in stable liposomes and their enhanced antipyretic effect. *Asian J. Pharm*, 3(3), 257-260.

[11] Goyal, A., Kumar, S., Nagpal, M., Singh, I., & Arora, S. (2011). Potential of Novel Drug Delivery Systems for Herbal Drugs. *Ind J Pharm Edu Res,* 45(3), 225-235.

[12] Egbaria, K. & Weiner, N. (1990) Liposomes as a topical drug delivery system, *Advanced Drug Delivery Reviews,* 5(1), 287-300.

[13] Kulkarni, P. R., Yadav, J. D. &, Vaidya, A. K. (2010). Liposomes: A Novel Drug Delivery System, *Int J Curr Pharm Res,* 3(2), 10-18.

[14] Kozubek, A., Gubernator, J., Przeworska, E. & Stasiuk, M. (2000). Liposomal drug delivery, a novel approach. *PLARosomes_,actq biochimica polonica,* 47(3), 639-649.

[15] Touitou, E., Junginger, H. E., Weiner, N. D. & Mezei, M. (1992). Liposomes as carriers for topical and transdermal delivery. *J. Pharm. Sci.,* 9(1),1189–1203.

[16] Schreier, H. & Bouwstra, J. A. (1994). Liposomes and niosomes as topical drug carriers: dermal and transdermal drug delivery. *J Control Rel,* 30, 1– 15.

[17] Nazzal, S., Smalyukh, I. I., Lavrentovich, O. D., & Khan, M. A. (2002). Preparation and *in vitro* characterization of a eutectic based semisolid self nanoemulsified drug delivery system of ubiquinone: mechanism and progress of emulsion formation. *Int J Pharm,* 235, 247-265.

[18] Kumar, M., Ahuja, M., & Sharma, S. K. (2008). Hepatoprotective study of curcumin soya lecithin complex. *Scientica Pharmaceutica,* 76, 761-774.

[19] Akbarzadeh, A., Rogaie, R., Joo S. W. et al. (2013). Liposome: classification, preparation, and applications. *Anoscale Research Letters*. 2013, 8:102,2-9.

[20] Kant Shashi, Kumar S. and Bhara P. (2012). A Complete Review On Liposomes. *International Research Journal of Pharmacy*. 3 (7), 10-16.

[21] Dua J. S., Rana, A. C. & Bhandari, A. K. (2012). Liposome: Methods of Preparation and Applications. *International Journal of Pharmaceutical Studies and Research*. 3 (2), 14-20.

[22] Mozafari, M. R., Johnson, C., Hatziantoniou, S. & Demetzos, C. (2008). "Nanoliposomes and their applications in food nanotechnology," *Journal of Liposome Research*, 18(1), 309-327.

[23] Laouini, A., Jaafar-Maalej, C., Sfar S. & Charcosset, C. (2012). Preparation, Characterization and Applications of Liposomes: State of the Art. *Journal of Colloid Science and Biotechnology*, 1(1), 147–168.

Chapter 4

NANOPARTICLES

1. INTRODUCTION

Nanoparticles are defined as particulate dispersions or solid particles with a size range of 10-1000nm. The drug is dissolved, entrapped, encapsulated, or attached to a nanoparticle matrix. Depending upon the method of preparation, nanoparticles, nanospheres, or nanocapsules can be obtained. Nanocapsules are systems in which the drug is confined to a cavity surrounded by a unique polymer membrane. At the same time, nanospheres are matrix systems in which the drug is physically and uniformly dispersed 55. According to the definition from NNI (National Nanotechnology Initiative), nanoparticles are structures of sizes ranging from 1 to 100 nm in at least one dimension. However, the prefix "nano" is commonly used for particles up to several hundred nanometers in size. Nanocarriers with optimized physicochemical and biological properties are taken up by cells more efficiently than larger ones. Liposome, solid lipids nanoparticles, dendrimers, polymers, silicon or carbon materials, and magnetic nanoparticles are examples of nanocarriers that have been tested as drug delivery systems (Figure 1) [1].

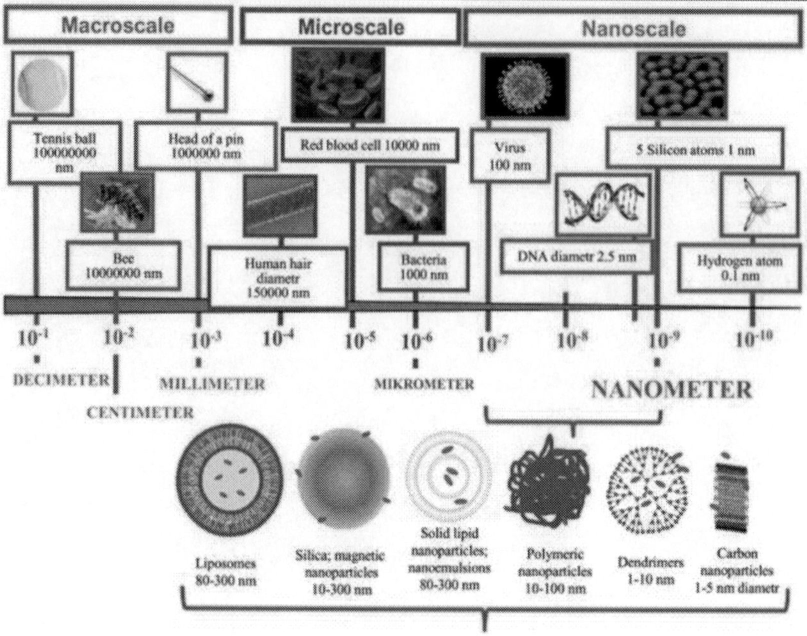
Macroscale
Microscale
Nanoscale
Tennis ball 100000000 nm
Head of a pin 1000000 nm
Red blood cell 10000 nm
Virus 100 nm
5 Silicon atoms 1 nm
Bee 10000000 nm
Human hair diametr 150000 nm
Bacteria 1000 nm
DNA diametr 2.5 nm
Hydrogen atom 0.1 nm
10-1
10-2
10-3
10-4
10-5
10-6
10-7
10-8
10-9
10-10
DECIMETER
CENTIMETER
MILLIMETER
MIKROMETER
NANOMETER
Liposomes 80-300 nm
Silica; magnetic nanoparticles 10-300 nm
Solid lipid nanoparticles; nanoemulsions 80-300 nm
Polymeric nanoparticles 10-100 nm
Dendrimers 1-10 nm
Carbon nanoparticles 1-5 nm diametr

Figure 1. Nanoparticles as a drug delivery.

Nanotechnology offers drugs in the nanometer size range, which enhances the performance in various dosage forms. Multiple advantages of nanosizing are mentioned below:

- Decreased fed/fasted variability
- Decreased patient-to-patient variability
- Enhanced solubility
- Increased oral bioavailability
- Increased rate of dissolution
- Increased surface area
- Less amount of dose required
- More rapid onset of therapeutic action

The primary goals in designing nanoparticles as a delivery system are to control particle size, surface properties, and release of pharmacologically active agents to achieve the drug's site-specific action at the therapeutically optimal rate and dose regimen. Though liposome has been used as potential carriers with unique advantages including protecting drugs from degradation, targeting to site of action and reduction toxicity or side effects, their applications are limited due to inherent problems such as low encapsulation efficiency, rapid leakage of the water-soluble drug in the presence of blood components and poor storage stability. On the other hand, polymeric nanoparticles offer some specific advantages over liposomes. For instance, they help increase the strength of drugs/proteins and possess useful controlled release properties [2-3].

1.1. Advantages of Nanoparticles

The benefits of using nanoparticles as a drug delivery system include the following:

1. Particle size and surface characteristics of nanoparticles can be easily manipulated to achieve passive and active drug targeting after parenteral administration.
2. They control and sustain the drug's release during the transportation and at the localization site, altering organ distribution of the drug and subsequent clearance of the drug to increase drug therapeutic efficacy and reduce side effects.
3. The choice of matrix constituents can readily modulate controlled release and particle degradation characteristics. Drug loading is relatively high, and drugs can be incorporated into the systems without any chemical reaction; this is an essential factor for preserving the drug activity.

4. Site-specific targeting can be achieved by attaching targeting ligands to the surface of particles or the use of magnetic guidance.
5. The system can be used for various administration routes, including oral, nasal, parenteral, intra-ocular, etc.

1.2. Disadvantages of Nanoparticles

1. The manufacturing costs of nanoparticle are high which result in overall product cost
2. Solvents are toxic which is used in the preparation process, Can start immune response and allergic reactions in the body,
3. Extensive use of poly (vinyl alcohol) as a stabilizer may have toxicity issues,
4. Nanoparticles are challenging to handle physically because particle-particle aggregation occurs due to their small size and large surface area [4].

2. Types of Nanoparticle

2.1. Liposome

Liposomes are concentric bilayered vesicles in which an aqueous volume is entirely enclosed by a membranous lipid bilayer mainly composed of natural or synthetic phospholipids. The liposome is characterized in terms of size, surface charge, and the number of bilayers. It exhibits several advantages in terms of amphiphilic character, biocompatibility, and ease of surface modification rendering it a suitable candidate delivery system for biotech drugs. Liposomes have been used successfully in the field of biology, biochemistry, and medicine since their origin. These alter the pharmacokinetic profile of loaded medications to a great extent, especially in proteins and peptides, and can be easily modified by surface attachment of polyethene glycol-units (PEG) stealth liposome and thus increase its circulation half-life [5].

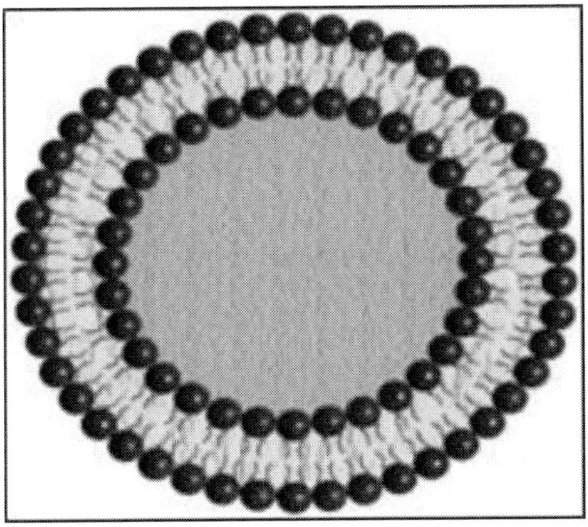

Figure 2. Liposome.

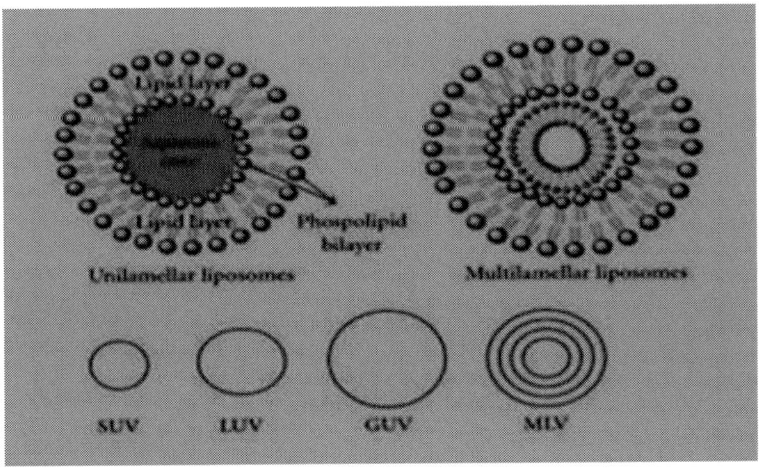
Lipid layer
Lipid layer
Phospholipid bilayer
Unilamellar liposomes
Multilamellar liposomes
SUV
LUV
GUV
MLV

Figure 3. Types of liposome.

Depending upon on their size and number of bilayers, they are classified into three basic types:

- *Multilamellar vesicles.* These vesicles consist of several lipid bilayers separated from one another by aqueous spaces. These entities are heterogeneous in size, often ranging from a few hundred to thousands of nanometers in diameter.
- *Small unilamellar vesicles.* Small unilamellar vesicles consist of a single bilayer surrounding the entrapped aqueous space having a size range of less than 100 nm.
- *Large unilamellar vesicles.* These vesicles consist of a single bilayer covering the tangled aqueous area having diameters larger than 100 nm.

2.2. Solid Lipid Nanoparticles

Solid lipid nanoparticles (SLN) were developed at the beginning of the 1990s as an alternative carrier system to emulsions, liposomes, and polymeric nanoparticles as a colloidal carrier system for controlled drug delivery. The main reason for their development is the combination of advantages from different carrier systems like liposome and polymeric nanoparticles. SLN has been developed and investigated for parenteral, pulmonary, and dermal application routes. Stable Lipid Nanoparticles consist of a solid lipid matrix, where the drug is customarily incorporated, with an average diameter below one μm. To avoid the aggregation and to stabilize the dispersion, different surfactants are used that have an accepted GRAS (Generally Recognized as Safe) status. SLN has been considered as new transfection agents using cationic lipids for the matrix lipid composition. Cationic solid lipid nanoparticles (SLN) for gene transfer can be formulated using the same cationic lipids for liposomal transfection agents [6].

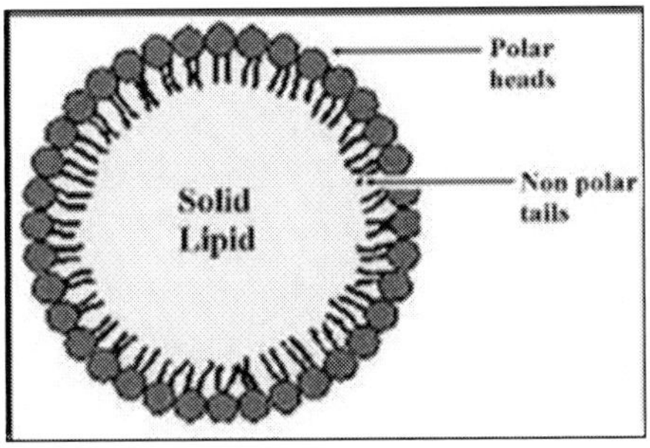
Polar heads
Non polar tails
Solid Lipid

Figure 4. Solid lipid nanoparticles.

2.3. Polymeric Nanoparticles

In comparison to SLN or nanosuspensions polymeric nanoparticles (PNPs) consists of a biodegradable polymer. The advantages of using PNPs in drug delivery are many. The most important is that they generally increase thc stability of any volatile pharmaceutical agents and that they are quickly and cheaply fabricated in large quantities by many methods. Also, polymeric nanoparticles may have engineered specificity, allowing them to deliver a higher pharmaceutical agent concentration to the desired location [7]. Polymeric nanoparticles are a broad class comprised of both vesicular systems (nanocapsules) and matrix systems (nanospheres).

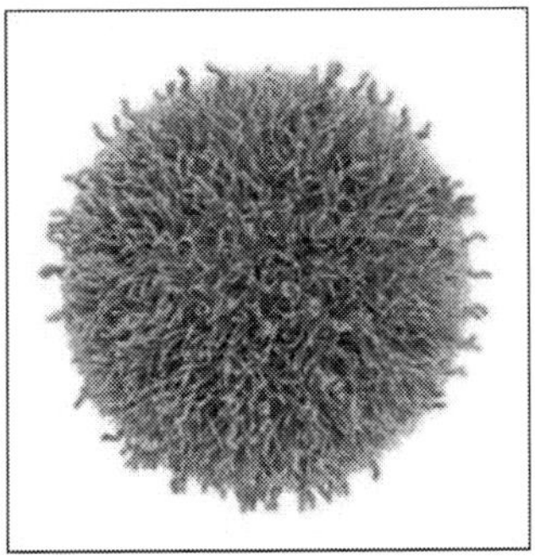

Figure 5. Polymeric nanoparticles.

2.4. Nanocapsules

Nanocapsules are systems in which the drug is confined to a cavity surrounded by a unique polymeric membrane. In contrast, nanospheres are systems in which the drug is dispersed throughout the polymer matrix. The various natural polymers like gelatin, albumin, and alginate are used to prepare the nanoparticles; however, they have some inherent disadvantages like low batch too- batch reproducibility, prone to degradation, and potential antigenicity. Synthetic polymers used for nanoparticle preparation may be in the form of preformed polymers, e.g., polyesters like polycaprolactone (PCL), polylactic acid (PLA) monomers that can be polymerized in situ, e.g., poly alkyl cyanoacrylate. The candidate drug is dissolved, entrapped, attached, or encapsulated throughout or within the polymeric shell/matrix. Depending on the method of preparation, the release characteristic of the incorporated drug can be controlled. Polymeric nanoparticulate systems are attractive modules for intracellular and site-specific delivery. Nanoparticles can be made to reach a target site under their size and surface modification with a specific recognition ligand. Their surface can be easily modified and functionalized [8-9].

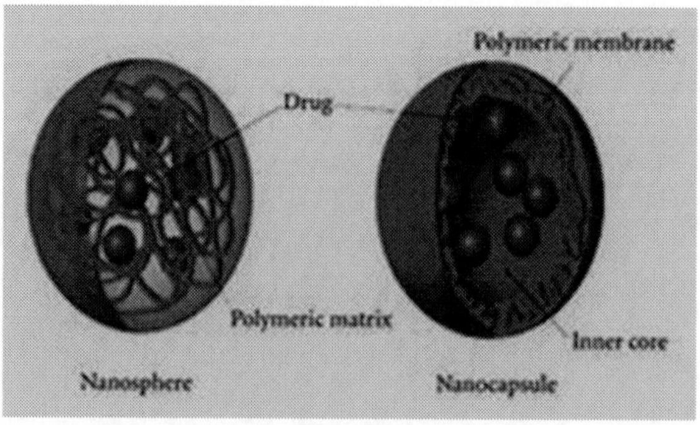
Polymeric membrane
Drug
Polymeric matrix
Inner core
Nanosphere
Nanocapsule

Figure 6. Nanosphere and nanocapsule.

2.5. Nanospheres

From its definition, nanospheres are considered as a matrix system in which the matrix is uniformly dispersed. These are spherical vesicular systems.

2.6. Dendrimers

Dendrimers, a unique polymers class, are highly branched macromolecules whose size and shape can be precisely controlled. Dendrimers are fabricated from monomers using either or divergent step-growth polymerization. The well-defined structure, monodispersity of length, surface functionalization capability, and stability are dendrimers' properties that make them attractive drug carrier candidates. Drug molecules can be incorporated into dendrimers via either complexation or encapsulation. Dendrimers are being investigated for drug and gene delivery, as carriers for penicillin, and in anticancer therapy [10].

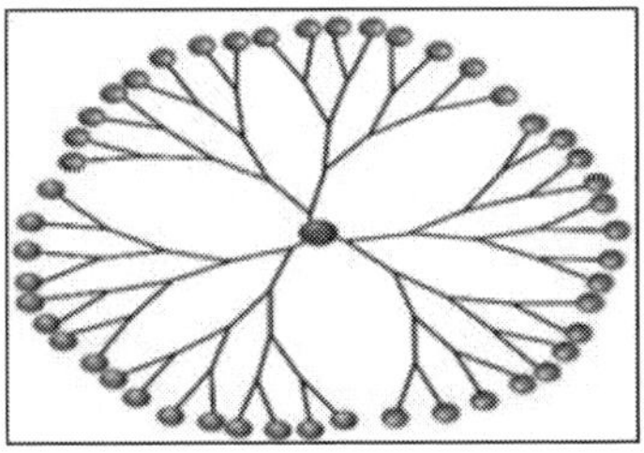

Figure 7. Dendrimers.

2.7. Nanotube

Carbon nanotubes (CNTs, also known as buckytubes) are allotropes of carbon with a cylindrical nanostructure. Nanotubes have been constructed with a length-to-diameter ratio of up to 132,000,000:1, which is significantly larger than any other material. These cylindrical carbon molecules have novel properties that make them potentially useful in many applications in nanotechnology, electronics, optics, and other fields of materials science and potential uses in architectural areas. They may also have applications in the construction of body armour. They exhibit extraordinary strength and unique electrical properties and are efficient thermal conductors [11-12].

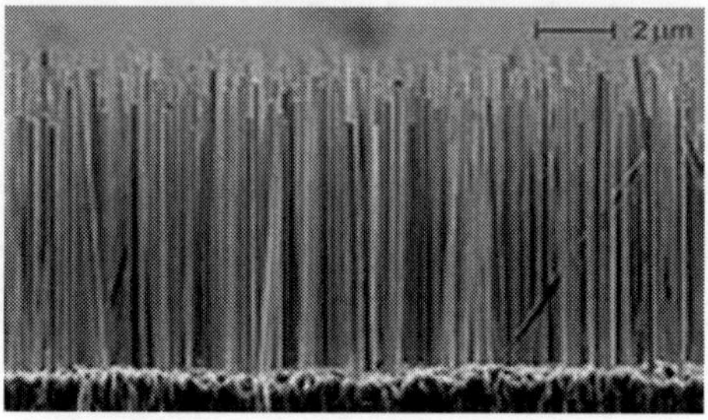
2 µm

Figure 8. Nanotubes.

2.8. Nanowire

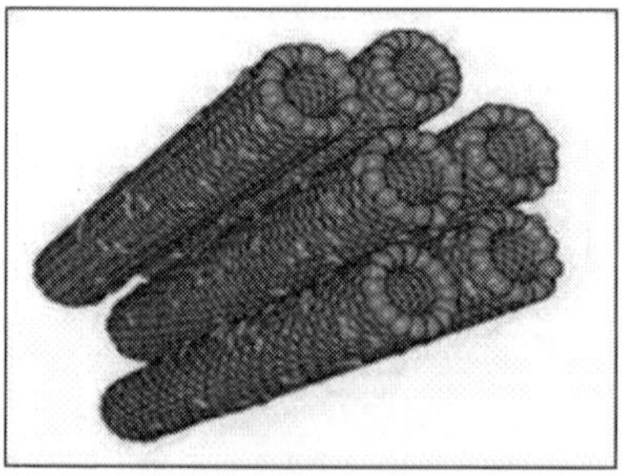

Figure 9. Nanowires.

A nanowire is a nanostructure with a diameter of a nanometer's order (10−9 meters). Alternatively, nanowires can be defined as structures with a thickness or diameter constrained to tens of nanometers or less and an unconstrained length. At these scales, quantum mechanical effects are significant — which coined the term "quantum wires." Many different types of nanowires exist, including metallic (e.g., Ni, Pt, Au), semiconducting (e.g., Si, InP, GaN, etc.), and insulating (e.g., SiO_2, TiO_2) [13].

2.9. Nanocrystals

Nanocrystal is any nanomaterial with at least one dimension ≤ 100nm, and that is single crystalline. More appropriately, any material with a size of less than 1 micrometre, i.e., 1000 nanometers, should be referred to as a nanoparticle, not a nanocrystal. For example, any particle that exhibits crystallinity regions should be termed nanoparticle or nanocluster based on dimensions. These materials are of substantial technological interest since many of their electrical and thermodynamic properties show strong size dependence and controlled through careful manufacturing processes.

Crystalline nanoparticles are also of interest because they often provide single-domain crystalline systems that can be studied to provide information that can help explain the behaviour of macroscopic samples of similar materials without the complicating presence of grain boundaries and other defects [14].

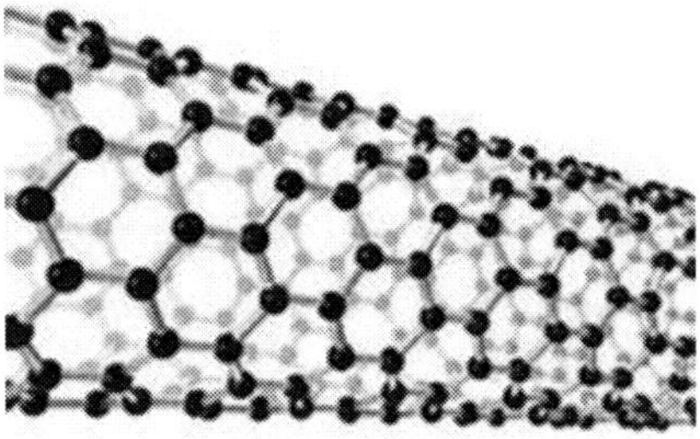

Figure 10. Nanocrystal.

2.10. Magnetic Nanoparticles

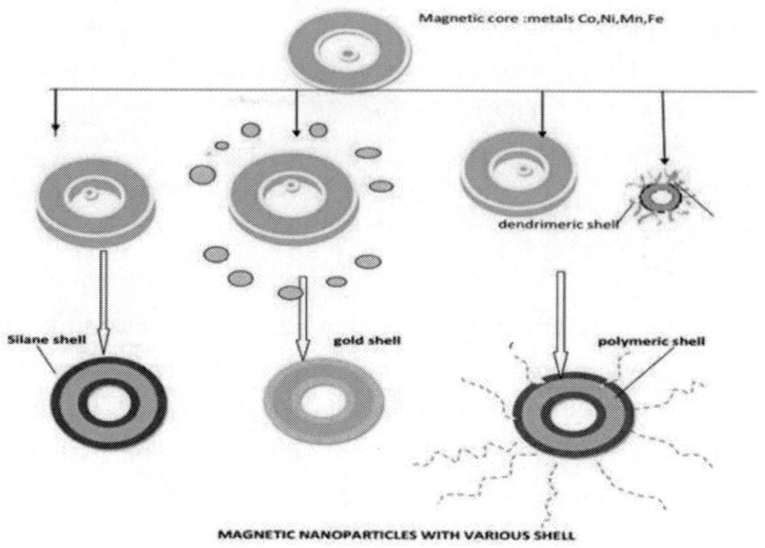
Magnetic core :metals Co,Ni,Mn,Fe
dendrimeric shell
Silane shell
gold shell
polymeric shell
MAGNETIC NANOPARTICLES WITH VARIOUS SHELL

Figure 11. Magnetic nanoparticles.

Magnetic nanoparticles exhibit a wide variety of attributes, which make them highly promising carriers for drug delivery. In particular, these are easy handling with the aid of an external magnetic field, the possibility of using passive and active drug delivery strategies, the ability of visualization (MNPs are used in MRI), and enhanced uptake by the target tissue resulting ineffective treatment at the therapeutically optimal doses [15]. However, in most cases where magnetic nanocarriers have been used, difficulties in achieving these objectives appeared. It is most likely associated with inappropriate features of magnetic nanoparticles or an inadequate magnet system. For instance, magnetic nanoparticles tend to aggregate into more massive clusters losing the specific properties connected with their small dimensions and making physical handling difficult. In turn, the magnetic force may not be strong enough to overcome the power of blood flow and to accumulate magnetic drugs only at the target site; therefore, designing magnetic drug delivery systems requires taking into consideration many factors, e.g., magnetic properties and size of particles, the strength of the magnetic field, drug loading capacity, the place of accessibility of target tissue, or the rate of blood flow [16]. Depending on magnetic properties, MNPs can be divided into pure metals (such as cobalt, nickel, manganese, and iron), their alloys, and oxides.

3. Preparation of Nanoparticles

The selection of the appropriate method for nanoparticle preparation depends on the polymer's physicochemical character and the drug to be loaded. Nanoparticles can be prepared from a variety of materials such as proteins, polysaccharides, and synthetic polymers. The selection of matrix materials is dependent on many factors, including [17].

Three methods have usually prepared nanoparticles:

- Macromolecule cross-linking
  - Heat cross-linking
  - Chemical cross-linking
- Polymerization based methods
  - Polymerization of the monomer
  - Emulsion (micellar) polymerization
  - Dispersion polymerization
  - Interfacial condensation polymerization
  - Interfacial complexation
- Polymerization of monomers
- Solvent extraction/evaporation
- Solvent displacement(nanoprecipitation)
- Salting out

4. Application of Nanoparticles

- These are used in intracellular targeting of anti-infective to reduce the difficulty to treat intracellular infections in the human body, e.g., ampicillin to nanoparticles for intra-bacterial infections
- To reduce the toxicity and increases the therapeutic activity of cytostatic drugs
- To improve the bioavailability and solubility of poorly soluble drugs
- To deliver medicine across the blood-brain barrier
- They are used as stable lipid nanoparticles in skin and hair care [18].

4.1. Application of Nanoparticles in Pharmaceutical Field

4.1.1. Nanoparticles as a Drug Delivery System for Peptides and Proteins

Large numbers of new therapeutic proteins and peptides are being discovered. Thus protein drug delivery technologies are of ever-increasing importance. Traditionally, the protein is delivered parenterally via solutions that are injected subcutaneously, intramuscularly, and intravenously. Although such injections benefit from high bioavailability, they fail to provide sustained plasma concentrations and suffer poor patient compliance due to the required frequency of injections. NPDDSs are designed to give the drug release over an extended period, minimizing the need for frequent injections. These can be used for systemic or oral delivery, and the biodegradable nature of the nanoparticulate materials alleviates the need for surgical removal [30]. To overcome the gastrointestinal barrier, the drug can be delivered in a colloidal carrier system (nanoparticles), which can potentially enhance the drug delivery system's interaction mechanisms and the epithelial cells in the GI tract. Nanoparticles based targeting epithelial cells using ligands is a potential strategy to improve nanoparticles' interaction with adsorptive enterocytes and M-cells of Peyer's patches in the GI tract [19].

Delivery routes and novel technologies for therapeutic peptides and proteins are:

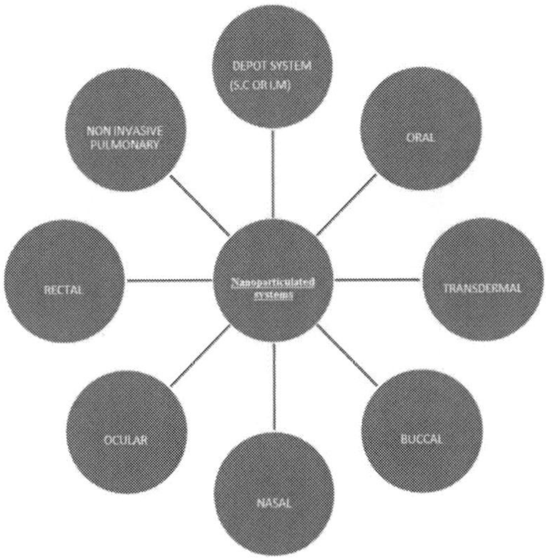
DEPOT SYSTEM
(S.C OR I.M)
NON INVASIVE
PULMONARY
ORAL
RECTAL
Nanoparticulated
systems
TRANSDERMAL
OCULAR
BUCCAL
NASAL

Figure 12. Nanoparticulated system.

4.1.2. Tumor Targeting Delivery Systems

The rationale for using nanoparticles for tumour targeting is based on the following characteristics:

- Nanoparticles will deliver a concentrated dose of the drug in the vicinity of the tumour targets via the enhanced permeability and retention effect or active targeting by ligands on the surface of nanoparticles.
- Nanoparticles will reduce the drug exposure of healthy tissues by limiting drug distribution to target organs [20].

Table 1. Various characteristics and brief application of nanosystem

Types of nanosystems	Size(nm)	Characteristics	Application
Carbon nanotubes	0.5-3 diameter and 20-100 length	Third allotropic crystalline form of carbon sheets either single layer (SWNT) or multi-layer(MWNT)	Functionalization enhanced solubility, to cell cytoplasm and nucleus, as a carrier for gene delivery, peptide delivery
Dendrimer	<10	Highly branched, nearly monodisperse polymer system produced by controlled polymerization; three central parts core, branch, and surface	Long circulatory, controlled delivery of bioactive, targeted delivery of bioactive to macrophages, liver targeting
Liposome	50-100	Phospholipid vesicles, biocompatible, versatile, good entrapment efficiency, offer easy	Long circulatory, offer passive and active delivery of gene, protein, peptide and various others
Metallic nanoparticles	<100	Gold and silver colloids, minimal size resulting in high surface area available for functionalization, stable	Drug and gene delivery, highly sensitive diagnostic assays, thermal ablation, and radiotherapy enhancement
Nanocrystals Quantum dots	2-9.5	Semiconducting material synthesized with II-VI and III-V column element, size between 10 and 100 A; bright fluorescence, narrow emission, broad UV excitation	The long term multiple colour imaging of liver cell; DNA; hybridization, immunoassay;receptor-mediated endocytosis, labelling of breast cancer marker HeR2 surface of cancer cells
Polymeric micelles	10-100nm	Block amphiphilic copolymer micelles, high drug entrapment	Long circulatory, target specific active and passive delivery, the diagnostic value
Polymeric nanoparticles	10-1000	Biodegradable, biocompatible, offer complete drug protection	Excellent carrier for controlled and sustained delivery of drugs .stealth and surface-modified nanoparticles can be used for passive and active delivery of bioactive

4.1.3. Nanoparticles in Dermatology

Concerning dermatological and transdermal therapy, the precise quantity of active ingredients necessary to achieve a given response cannot be predicted with certainty. This lack of precision is primarily due to the variability of skin penetration by the active ingredient related to the thickness of the epidermis and its keratin layer and the mechanical removal of the applied formulation if a dressing does not cover the affected area. To overcome many of these drawbacks mentioned above, attempts have been made to introduce lipid nanoparticles into the cosmetic and pharmaceutical fields. Solid lipid nanoparticles (SLNs) and nanostructured lipid carriers (NLC) (3) are novel colloidal delivery systems with many decorative and dermatological features, such as adhesive properties when applied to the skin. These properties bring many other advantages, such as occlusion and skin hydration, absorption-increasing effects, active penetration enhancement, and controlled-release properties [21].

4.1.4. Nanoparticle in Cosmetics

The present review aims to study a promising area of Nanoparticles used in various cosmetic products like Deodorant, Soap, Toothpaste, Shampoo, Hair conditioner, Anti-wrinkle cream, Foundation, Face powder, Lipstick, Blush, Eye shadow, Nail polish, Perfume, and After-shave lotion, etc. In particular, NLCs have been identified as a potential next-generation cosmetic delivery agent that can provide enhanced skin hydration, bioavailability, agent's stability, and controlled occlusion [22].

References

[1] Martin C. R. Welcome to nanomedicine. *Nanomedicine*. 2006; 1(1):5.

[2] V. Sankar, S. Ramesh, V. Shanmugam, *A Textbook of novel drug delivery systems* :1.

[3] The Royal Society. *Nanoscience and nanotechnologies: opportunities and uncertainties*. London: Royal Society, 2004:4.

[4] Suri SS, Fenniri H, Singh B: Nanotechnology-based drug delivery systems. *J Occup Med Toxicol*.

[5] Vila A, Sanchez A, Tobio M, Calvo P, Alonso MJ. Design of biodegradable particles for protein delivery. *J Control Release* 2002; 78: 15-24.

[6] Mu L, Feng SS. A novel controlled release formulation for the anticancer drug paclitaxel (Taxol(R)): PLGA nanoparticles containing vitamin E TPGS. *J Control Release* 2003; 86: 33-48.

[7] Venkatesan, P., V. SreeJanardha nan, C. Muralidharan, and K. Valliappan. *Acta Chim. Slov*., 2012; 59: 242–248.

[8] KannappanValliappan, Sree Janardhanan Vaithiyanathan and Venkatesan Palanivel. *Chromatographia*, 2013; 76(5): 287-292

[9] Redhead, H. (1997). "*Drug loading of biodegradable nanoparticles for site-specific drug delivery*". University of Nottingham Nottingham.

[10] http://www.nano.irS.

[11] http://www.nanotechnologydevelopment.com/products/introductio n-to- nanoparticles.html.

[12] http://www.nanotechproject.org/inventories/medicine/.

[13] http://www.yashnanotech.com/nano-application.php.

[14] http://www.understandingnano.com/medicine.html.

[15] Jain S., Jain N.K. Liposomes as a drug carrier, In Jain NK, editor. *Controlled and novel drug delivery*. 2nded. CBS publisher, New Delhi, 2002,.304-52.

[16] Baba R. Patent and Nanomedicine. *Nanomedicine* (2007) 2(3), 351-374.

[17] Khopde AJ, Jain, NK. Dendrimer as potential delivery system for bioactive In: Jain NK, editor. *Advances in controlled and novel drug delivery*. CBS publisher, New Delhi, 2001, 361-80.

[18] P. Venkatesan et al. / *International Journal on Pharmaceutical and Biomedical Research* (*IJPBR*) Vol. 2(3), 2011, 107-117.

[19] Sathiya Sundar, R., Murugesan, A., Venkatesan, P. and Manavalan, R. Formulation Development and Evaluation of Carprofen Microspheres. *Int. J. Pharm Tech Research*. 2010 Vol. 2, No. 3, 1674-1676.

[20] Venkatesan, P., Manavalan R.and Valliappan, K. Microencapsulation: A Vital Technique In Novel Drug Delivery System. *J. Pharm. Sci. & Res*. Vol. 1(4), 2009, 26-35

[21] Hussain N, Jani PU, Florence AT. Enhanced oral uptake of tomato lectin-conjugated nanoparticles in the rat. *Pharm Res* 1997; 14: 613-8.

[22] Arunkumar et al.,: Formulation, Evaluation and Optimization of Sustained Release Bilayer tablets of Niacin and Green Tea extract by employing Box-Behnken design, *J. Sci. Res. Phar.,* 2016; 5(2): 23.

[23] Arunkumar et al.,: Development and Validation of New Analytical methods for Simultaneous estimation of Epigallocatechin gallate, a component of Green Tea extractand Niacin in a Pharmaceutical dosage form, *J. Pharm. Res*., 2016; 5(2): 21-24.

[24] Cao Q., Han X., Li L. Enhancement of the efficiency of magnetic targeting for drug delivery: Development and evaluation of magnet system. *J Magn Magn Mater*, 2011,323, 1919–1924.

[25] Pangi Z., Beletsi A., Evangelatos K. PEG-ylated nanoparticles for biological and pharmaceutical application. *Adv Drug Del Rev*. 2003; 24:403–19.

[26] Scholes P. D., Coombes A. G., Illum L., Davis S. S., Wats J. F., Ustariz C., Vert M., Davies M. C. Detection and determination of surface levels of poloxamer and PVA surfactant on biodegradable nanospheres using SSIMS and XPS. *J Control Release*. 1999; 59:261–78.

[27] Kreuter J. Physicochemical characterization of polyacrylic nanoparticles. *Int J Pharm*. 1983; 14:43–58.

[28] Magenhein B, Levy MY, Benita S. A new *in vitro* technique for the evaluation of drug release profile from colloidal carriers ultrafi ltration technique at low pressure. *Int J Pharm*. 1993; 94:115–23.

[29] Kreuter J. Nanoparticles. In: Kreuter J, editor. *Colloidal drug delivery systems*. New York: Marcel Dekker; 1994. p. 219–342.

[30] Kwon H. Y., Lee J. Y., Choi S. W., Jang .Y, Kim J. H. Preparation of PLGA nanoparticles containing estrogen by emulsification-diffusion method. *Colloids Surf A Physicochem Eng Aspects*. 2001; 182:123.

Chapter 5

HYDROGEL

1. INTRODUCTION

Hydrogels are a unique, three-dimensional (3D) viscoelastic network composed of hydrophilic polymers cross-linked through intermolecular or intramolecular forces of attraction, which permits the diffusion attachment of molecules and cells. Hydrogels can absorb many liquid fluids and swell readily without dissolving, exhibiting an intermediate behaviour between solid and liquid material. The swelling properties are due to the high thermodynamical affinity that hydrogel has for the solvent itself. It has high versatility and increased ability. For shape and mechanical strength, these hydrogel networks establish equilibrium with their surroundings' liquid and temperature [1].

Hydrogels can be prepared from water-soluble polymer, encompassing a wide range of chemical composition and bulk physical properties. The hydrogel is sometimes found as a colloidal gel in which water is the dispersion medium. The hydrogel can contain over 90% water. Formulation of hydrogels can be prepared in various physical forms, including slabs, nanoparticles, microparticles, coatings, and films [2].

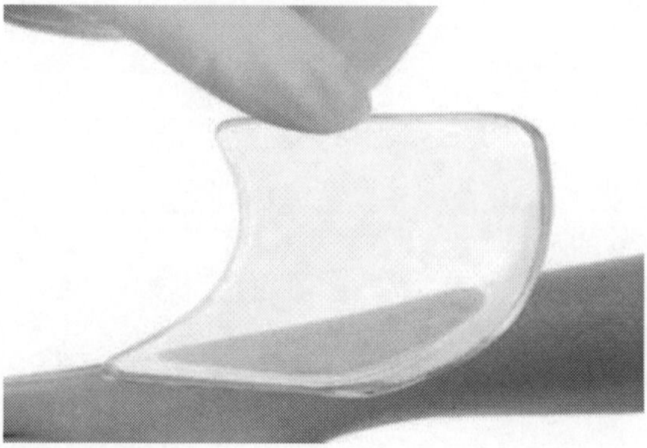

Figure 1. Hydrogel.

Hydrogels can retain a large amount of water within their structures, making the design rubbery, which resembles the living tissue. Hydrogels are soft, and because of the three-dimensional hydrophilic polymeric networks, it results in high biocompatibility [3]. Biomedical applications such as cell therapeutics, wound healing, cartilage/bone regeneration, and the sustained release of drugs, tissue adhesives, tissue engineering scaffolds, drug delivery carriers biosensors, and soft robotic and electronic components are due to their biocompatibility and the similarity of their physical properties to natural tissues. In response to different stimuli such as temperature, pH, light, ionic strength, electric or magnetic field, and chemicals, hydrogels can exhibit unusual changes in their swelling behaviour, network structure, mechanical properties, and volume phase transitions, resulting in an enormous potential for various advanced technological applications [4]. The unique physical properties of hydrogels have gained attention towards their use in drug delivery applications. Their highly porous structure can easily be tuned by controlling the density of cross-links in the gel matrix and the hydrogels' affinity for the aqueous environment in which they are swollen. The porosity of hydrogel also permits the loading of drugs into the gel matrix and subsequent drug release, which depends on the small molecules or macromolecules' diffusion coefficient through the gel network. Indeed, the benefit of hydrogels for drug delivery may be largely pharmacokinetics. Specifically, a depot formulation is created from which drugs slowly elute, maintaining a high local concentration of medicine in the surrounding tissues over an extended period. However, they can also be used for systemic delivery. Hydrogels can be used in the peritoneum and other sites *in vivo*. Hydrogels may be chemically stable, or they may degrade and eventually disintegrate and dissolve. Biodegradability or dissolution may be designed into hydrogels via enzymatic, hydrolytic, or environmental (e.g., pH, temperature, or electric field) pathways. Degradation is not always desirable; it depends on the drug delivery device's time scale and location. They are relatively deformable and can conform to the shape of the surface to which they are applied. At the site of application, when the body is not horizontal, the mucoadhesive and bioadhesive properties of some hydrogel can be advantageous in immobilizing them at that site [5]. Hydrogel dressings provide more excellent safety as compared to traditional sauces. It can absorb physiological exudates from wounds. It enhances wound healing by providing a moisture balance around the damage. Hydrogels should possess anti-infection properties. Hydrogel dressing gives antibacterial activity by the following two approaches- The first approach is to introduce the antibacterial agent to the hydrogel matrix. Titanium dioxide (TiO_2) has a unique capability in the photocatalytic bacterial disruption. It can self-clean and remove a broad spectrum of pollutants. It has been reported that the antibacterial activity has improved by taking photo-catalysts into materials for wound dressings. The TiO_2 and curcumin were incorporated into the hydrogel made of sodium alginate (SA) and polyvinyl alcohol (PVA); the combination showed antibacterial activity against Gram-Positive and Gram-Negative bacterium.

Another way to prepare antibacterial hydrogel is by using antibacterial materials as a hydrogel matrix. The anti-bacterial activity of the dressing material has been improved by taking photo-catalysts into materials for wound dressings. Products constructed from chitin and its derivatives are biomass materials with antimicrobial activity [6].

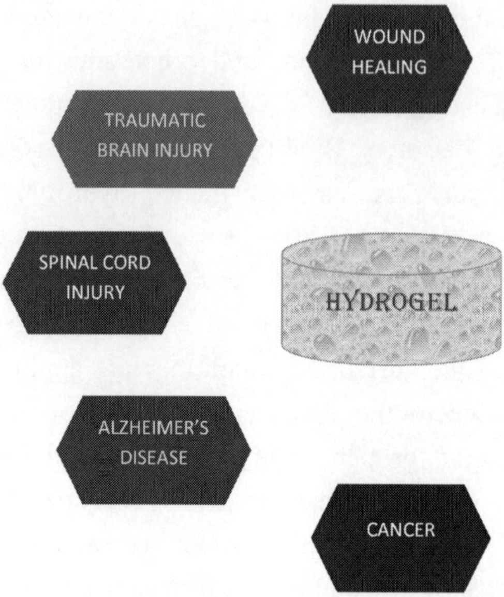
WOUND HEALING
TRAUMATIC BRAIN INJURY
CUTANEOUSLEI SHMANIASIS
SPINAL CORD INJURY
HYDROGEL
BREAST IMPLANTS
ALZHEIMER'S DISEASE
PARKINSON'S DISEASE
CANCER

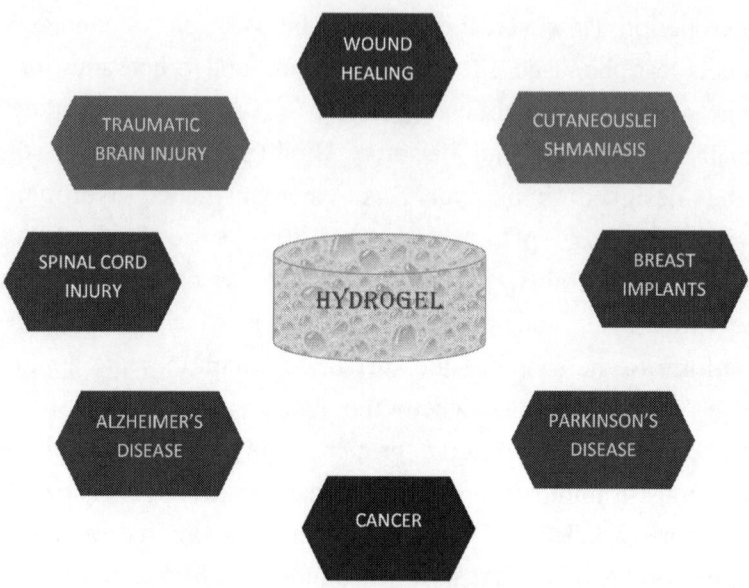

Figure 2. Hydrogels are used to cure various disorders such as Wounds.

2. Classification

The hydrogel products can be classified on different bases as detailed below:

2.1. Classification based on source

Hydrogels can be classified into two groups based on their natural or synthetic origins

a. *Natural hydrogels* - Natural hydrogels are biodegradable, biocompatible, and good cell adhesion properties. Two major types of natural polymers are used to produce natural hydrogels are proteins such as collagen, gelatin and, lysozyme (LYZ) and polysaccharides such as hyaluronic acid (HA) and alginate and Chitosan (Cts).
b. *Synthetic hydrogels* - They are more useful than natural hydrogels because they can be engineered to have a much more comprehensive range of mechanical and chemical properties than their wild counterparts. Polyethene glycol (PEG) based hydrogels are the widely used material in biomedical applications due to their nontoxicity, compatibility, and low immunogenicity.
c. *Hybrid hydrogels* - They are a combination of natural and synthetic polymer hydrogels. To combine the advantages of both synthetic and natural hydrogels, many naturally occurring biopolymers such as dextran, collagen, Chitosan have been combined with synthetic polymers such as poly (N-isopropyl acrylamide) and polyvinyl alcohol [7].

2.2. Classification According to the Polymeric Composition

a. *Homopolymeric hydrogels* - They are a basic structural unit comprising of any polymer network referred to as a polymer network derived from a single species of monomer. Depending on the nature of the monomer and polymerization technique, homopolymers may have a cross-linked skeletal structure. Homopolymers can be prepared using polyethene glycol dimethacrylate as a cross-linking agent, poly (2-hydroxyethyl methacrylate) (poly HEMA) monomer, and benzoin isobutyl ether as the UV-sensitive initiator. The film was prepared in de-ionized water and treated with UV radiation (λ = 253.7 nm, 11 mm distance from the source for 20 minutes). The film was then immersed for 24 h in water until it is fully saturated to remove toxic or unreacted substances that could damage living tissue. Besides contact lenses, they can also be applied in artificial skin manufacturing and burn dressings, ensuring the right wound-healing conditions. It is also used for bone marrow and spinal cord cell regeneration, scaffolds for promoting cell adhesion, and artificial cartilage production [8-9].

b. *Copolymeric hydrogels* are comprised of two or more different monomer species with at least one hydrophilic component, arranged in block or alternating configuration, a random, along the polymer network chain. Synthesized by polymerization of BLG N-carboxy anhydride, initiated by diamine groups located at the ends of poly (ethylene oxide) chains of the poloxamer, a thermoplastic co-polymeric hydrogel based on γ-benzyl L-glutamate (BLG) and poloxamer was formed. This hydrogel was pH and temperature-sensitive and characterized for drug delivery application [10].
c. *Multipolymer interpenetrating polymeric hydrogel (IPN),* an introductory hydrogels class, has a network system made of two independent cross-linked synthetic and natural polymer components. In the semi- IPN hydrogel, the one-piece is a cross-linked polymer, and the other piece is a non-cross-linked polymer. IPN method can overcome thermodynamic incompatibility due to the permanent interlocking of network segments, and limited phase separation can be obtained. The interlocked structure of the cross-linked IPN components is believed to ensure the bulk and surface morphology [11].

2.2.1. Advantages

a. Dense hydrogel matrices can be produced which feature stiffer and more rigid mechanical properties.
b. Controllable physical properties and more efficient drug loading compared to conventional hydrogels.
c. Drug loading is often performed in conjunction with the interpenetrating hydrogel phase [12].

2.3. According to the Biodegradable

a. *Biodegradable hydrogels* - Hydrogels are many biodegradable polymers created by nature biodegradable, such as Chitosan, fibrin, and agar. Poly (aldehyde guluronate), polyanhydrides, and poly (N-isopropyl acrylamide) are examples of synthetic biodegradable polymers.
b. *Non-biodegradable hydrogels* - Various vinylated monomers or macromers such as 2-hydroxyethyl methacrylate (HEMA), methoxyl poly (ethylene glycol) (MPEG), 2- hydroxypropyl methacrylate (HPMA), and acrylamide (AAm) are widely applied in the preparation of non-biodegradable hydrogels [13].

2.4. Classification Based on Configuration

The classification of hydrogels depends on their physical structure, and chemical composition can be classified as follows:

a. Amorphous (non-crystalline).
b. Semicrystalline: A complex mixture of amorphous and crystalline phases.
c. Crystalline.

2.5. Classification Based on the Type of Cross-Linking

Hydrogels can be divided into two categories based on the chemical or physical nature of the cross-link junctions.

a. Chemically cross-linked networks have permanent junctions.
b. Physical networks have transient junctions that arise from either polymer chain entanglements or physical interactions as hydrogen bonds or hydrophobic interactions [14].

2.6. Classification Based on Physical Appearance

Hydrogel's appearance as a matrix, film, or microsphere depends on the polymerization technique involved in the preparation process.

2.7. Classification According to Network Electrical Charge

Hydrogels may be categorized into four groups based on the presence or absence of electrical charge located on the cross-linked chains:

a. Nonionic (neutral).
b. Ionic (including anionic or cationic).
c. Amphoteric electrolyte (ampholytic) containing both acidic and basic groups.
d. Zwitterionic (polybetaines) containing both anionic and cationic groups [15].

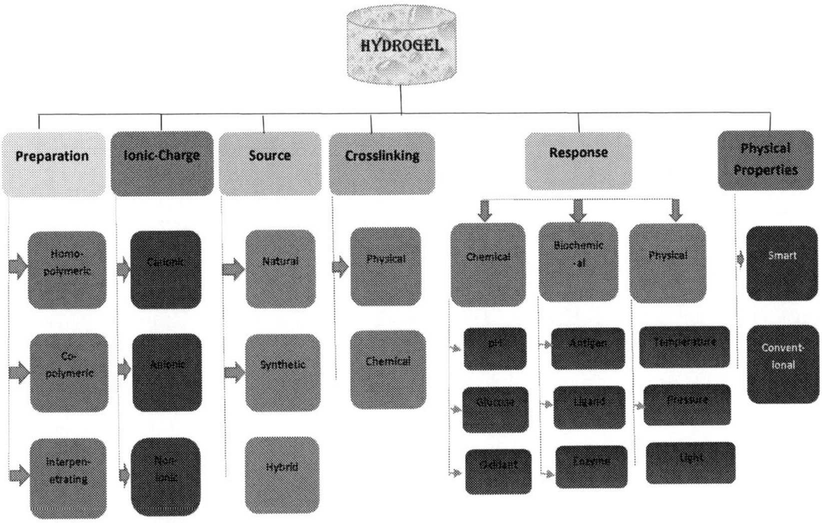
HYDROGEL
Preparation
Ionic-Charge
Source
Crosslinking
Response
Physical Properties
Homo-polymeric
Co-polymeric
Interpen-etrating
Natural
Synthetic
Hybrid
Physical
Chemical
Chemical
Biochemic-al
Physical
Smart
Convent-ional

Figure 3. Classification of hydrogels based on different properties.

3. PROPERTIES OF HYDROGEL

For any material, the physical, chemical, and mechanical properties play an essential role in determining if it is suitable for a given application. However, for hydrogels, these properties are highly dependent on environmental conditions as well. Thus, while choosing the properties of a hydrogel, mimicking the in situ conditions becomes imperative. Hydrogels have various properties, including their absorption capacity, swelling behaviour, permeability, surface properties, optical properties, and mechanical properties, making them promising materials for a wide variety of applications. The characteristics of the polymer chains and the cross-linking structures in these aqueous solutions play an essential role in the outcome of the hydrogel's properties [16].

3.1. Swelling and Absorption Capacity

The polymer chains in a hydrogel interact with the solvent molecule (usually water) and expand to the fully solvated state. At the same time, the cross-linked structure applies a retroactive force to pull the chains inside. Equilibrium is achieved when these expanding and retracting forces counterbalance each other. The swelling ratio or water content, given by Eq. 1 and Eq. 2, is generally used to describe hydrogels' swelling behaviour.

$$\text{Water content} = [\{\text{weight of water} \div (\text{weight of water} + \text{weight of gel})\} \times 100]$$

$$\text{Swelling ratio} = (\text{weight of swollen gel} \div \text{weight of dry gel})$$

The swelling characteristics are crucial to hydrogels in biomedical and pharmaceutical applications. The equilibrium swelling ratio influences the solute diffusion coefficient, surface wet ability and mobility, and the hydrogel's optical and mechanical properties. Many factors are determined by the swelling properties, including monomers' type and composition, cross-linking density, and other environmental factors such as temperature, pH, and ionic strength [17].

3.2. Porosity

Pores may be formed in hydrogels by phase separation during synthesis, or they may exist as smaller pores within the network. The average pore size, the pore size distribution, and the pore interconnections are essential factors of a hydrogel matrix that are often difficult to quantify and are usually included together in the parameter called "tortuosity." The sufficient diffusion path length across an HG film barrier is estimated by the film thickness times the pore volume fraction ratio divided by the tortuosity. In turn, these factors are most influenced by the composition and crosslink density of the hydrogel polymer network.

Pore-size distributions of hydrogels are strongly affected by three factors:

- The concentration of the polymer strands' chemical cross-links is determined by the initial ratio of cross-linker to monomer.
- The concentration of the polymer strands' physical entanglements is determined by the initial concentration of all polymerizable monomers in the aqueous solution.
- The polyelectrolyte hydrogel's net charge is determined by the initial concentration of the cationic and anionic monomer. [18].

3.3. Permeability of Hydrogels

Permeability is a hydrogel's ability to transmit another substance such as fluids, cells, or proteins. Developing hydrogel membranes and coatings of appropriate permeability characteristics is key to several bio-artificial organ transplantations' success. A hydrogel's permeability to water and solutes can be adjusted over a wide range by varying the cross-linker concentration at synthesis or copolymerizing with more hydrophilic or hydrophobic monomers [19]. Some of the real-life situations where the permeability of hydrogels is critical are oxygen permeation for contact lens applications, nutrient, and immunological bio-substance transport for immune-isolation and release of drugs and proteins for drug delivery systems.

3.4. Surface Properties of Hydrogel

Biocompatibility is a hydrogel's ability to reside in the body without inducing significant immune response or toxicity. The critical question in biocompatibility is how the hydrogel transduces its structural makeup to direct or influence proteins, cells, and organisms' response. This transduction occurs through the hydrogel's surface properties, i.e., the body reads the surface structure and responds to it. A hydrogel's surface can be rough, smooth, or stepped; it can be composed of different chemistries or highly crystalline, disordered, and inhomogeneous. Studies have been performed on the importance of roughness, wettability, surface mobility, chemical composition, crystallinity, and heterogeneity. However, significant research has not yet been conducted on determining which parameters are of utmost importance in understanding biological responses to surfaces. Some of the techniques used for determining the surface property include electron spectroscopy, secondary ion mass spectrometry, scanning electron microscopy, Fourier transforms infrared spectroscopy, scanning tunnelling microscopy, and atomic force microscopy. The information obtained using these methods can monitor contamination, ensure surface reproducibility, and explore the hydrogels' interaction with living systems [20].

3.5. Mechanical Properties of Hydrogels

The mechanical properties of hydrogels depend on their composition and structure. Because of the high water content of fully swollen hydrogels, they usually have weak mechanical strengths. The hydrogel's mechanical properties are affected by the co-monomer composition, crosslinking density, polymerization conditions, and swelling degree. The hydrogel's mechanical strength is often derived entirely from the cross-links in the system, particularly in the swollen state where physical entanglements are almost non-existent. The dependence of mechanical properties on crosslink density has been studied intensively by many researchers. However, it should be noted that when the crosslinking density is altered, changes to properties other than strength also occur. For example, increasing the cross-linker concentration would make the polymer chains closer, reducing the diffusivity, release, and swelling rates, including the maximum degree of swelling. The swelling would mean that these properties will need to be re-measured every time additional cross-links are added. Theories of elasticity and viscoelasticity best understand the mechanical behaviour of hydrogels. These theories are based on the time-independent and time-dependent recovery of the chain orientation and structure, respectively. Elasticity theory assumes that when stress is applied to the hydrogel, the strain response is instantaneous. However, for many biomaterials, including hydrogels and tissues, this is not a valid assumption. For example, if weight is suspended from a ligament specimen, the ligament continues to extend even though the load is constant.

Similarly, if the ligament is elongated to a fixed length, the load drops continuously with time. The ligament is due to creep and stress relaxation, respectively, and these are the result of viscous flow in the material. Despite this liquid-like behaviour, hydrogels are functionally solids and are thus assumed to be perfectly elastic for the present study. A brief introduction to the elastic theory's fundamentals is presented [21].

4. THEORY OF ELASTICITY

Elasticity is the physical property of a material by which it returns to its original shape after the force under which it deforms is removed.

The applied force is usually referred to as stress, the force acting per unit cross-sectional area of the material, while the relative deformation is called strain. The elastic regime is characterized by a linear relationship between stress and pressure. The ratio of stress to strain is constant for a given material and is the material's defining mechanical property. Whether the force applied is perpendicular or parallel to the area supporting it, the stresses and strains can be axial or shear. The proportionality constant for the axial stress ratio to the axial strain is called Young's modulus (represented by E).

In contrast, the shear stress ratio to shear strain is referred to as shear modulus (represented by G). A linearly, isotropic and homogenous material E and Gare sufficient to completely characterize the material's mechanical properties. However, most polymeric materials and tissue samples are anisotropic, meaning they have different properties in different directions. For example, bone, ligament, and sutures are stiffer in the longitudinal direction compared to the transverse direction. For such materials, more than two elastic constants must relate the stress and the strain properties on a macroscopic scale. However, on a microscopic scale, polymers are comparatively isotropic, and the flexible and shear modulus are adequate to characterize their local mechanical properties fully. In the next chapter, the construction of a microscope-based four magnet device will be presented. This device can be non-intrusively utilized to fully characterize hydrogels' local mechanical properties [22-23].

5. Methods of Preparation

Based on the methods of preparation, hydrogels may be classified as (1) homo-polymer (2) copolymer (3) Semi-interpenetrating network (4) interpenetrating network. Homo-polymer hydrogels are cross-linked networks of one type of hydrophilic monomer unit. In contrast, copolymer hydrogels are produced by cross-linking of two co-monomer teams, at least one of which must be hydrophilic to render them swellable. Finally, interpenetrating polymeric hydrogels are made by preparing a first network that is then swollen in a monomer. The latter reacts to form a second intermeshing network structure.

5.1. Homo-Polymeric Hydrogel

Homopolymers are referred to as polymer networks derived from single species of monomer. It is the basic structural unit and comprising of any polymer network. Homopolymers may have a cross-linked skeletal structure depending on the nature of the monomer and polymerization technique. Cross-linked homopolymers are used in the drug delivery system and contact lenses. The possible way of preparing homo-polymeric hydrogel film is poly (2-hydroxyethyl methacrylate) (poly HEMA) as a monomer, polyethene glycol dimethacrylate as a cross-linking agent, and benzoin isobutyl ether as the UV-sensitive initiator. The film was prepared in de-ionized water and treated with UV radiation (λ = 253.7 nm, 11 mm distance from the source for 20 minutes). The film was then immersed for 24 h in water until it is fully saturated to remove toxic or unreacted substances that could damage living tissue. Besides contact lenses, pHEMA can also be applied in artificial skin manufacturing and burn dressings, ensuring the right wound-healing conditions. It is also used for bone marrow and spinal cord cell regeneration, scaffolds for promoting cell adhesion, and artificial cartilage production. Another low molecular weight crosslinking agent used in poly HEMA hydrogel synthesis is 1, 1,1-trimethylolpropane trimethacrylate. The hydrogel obtained with this agent is soft and contains 30-40% of water & distinguished by its high oxygen permeability. These properties have translated its use in contact lenses as matrices for drug delivery systems and soft tissue implants. If the mechanical properties of the hydrogel are improved, its application could further be extended. Polyethene glycol (PEG) based hydrogels are responsive towards external stimuli, and hence these smart hydrogels are widely used in the drug delivery system. Chemically cross-linked PEG hydrogels are used as scaffolds for protein recombination and functional tissue production. It is a suitable biomaterial for the efficient and controlled release of drugs, proteins, biomolecules, and growth factors [23].

5.2. Co-Polymeric Hydrogel

Co-polymeric hydrogels are composed of two types of monomer in which at least one is hydrophilic. Synthesized the biodegradable triblock poly (ethylene glycol)-poly(εcaprolactone)- poly(ethylene glycol) (PECE) co-polymeric hydrogel for the development of a drug delivery system. The mechanism involves here is the ring-opening copolymerization of ε-caprolactone. In the triblock synthesis, mPEG was used as the initiator. The stannous octoate as the catalyst, and hexamethylene diisocyanate as a coupling agent. This co-polymeric block is capable of forming a hydrogel when it is applied in-situ. The study reveals that the hydrogel was biodegradable and bio-compatible. It could release both the hydrophobic and hydrophilic drugs, including proteins, over a sustained period [24].

5.3. Semi- Inter Penetrating Network (Semi-IPN)

If one polymer is linear and penetrates another cross-linked network without any other chemical bonds between them, it is called a semi-interpenetrating system. Semi-IPNs can more effectively preserve rapid kinetic response rates to pH or temperature due to the absence of restricting interpenetrating elastic network while still providing the benefits like modified pore size & slow drug release. The system contained both covalent and ionic bonds. The covalent bonds retained the three-dimensional hydrogel structure, and the ionic bonds imparted the hydrogel with higher mechanical strength and pH-responsive reversibility.

Semi-IPN of gum arabic and the crosslinked copolymer of pHEMA. The pHEMA synthesized in the presence of ammonium persulfate and N, Nmethylene bisacrylamide initiator and the crosslinking agent, respectively. The hydrogel was loaded with silver nanoparticles via in situ reductions of silver nitrate using trisodium citrate as a reducing agent. The hydrogel-stabilized silver nanoparticles showed excellent antibacterial properties [24].

5.4. Inter Penetrating Network (IPN)

IPNs are conventionally defined as an intimate combination of two polymers, at least one of which is synthesized or cross-linked in the other's immediate presence. The IPNs is typically done by immersing a pre-polymerized hydrogel into a solution of monomers and a polymerization initiator. IPN method can overcome thermodynamic incompatibility due to the permanent interlocking of network segments, and limited phase separation can be obtained. The interlocked structure of the cross-linked IPN components is believed to ensure the bulk and surface morphology stability. The main advantages of IPNs are relatively dense hydrogel matrices that can be produced, which feature stiffer and more rigid mechanical properties, controllable physical properties, and more efficient drug loading compared to conventional hydrogels. Drug loading is often performed in conjunction with the polymerization of the interpenetrating hydrogel phase. IPN pore sizes and surface chemistries can also be controlled to tune the drug release kinetics, interaction between the hydrogel and the surrounding tissues, and its mechanical properties. Interpenetrating phases with different degradation profiles and different swelling responses to physiological conditions can provide multiple controls over hydrogels' swelling responses and thus the drug release kinetics. IPNs can moderate the effect of environmental changes on hydrogel responses and hence drug burst release because of their ability to restrict the equilibrium swelling of either or both of the interpenetrating phases according to the elasticity (i.e., crosslinking density) [25].

REFERENCES

[1] Ehterami Arian, Salehi Majid, Farzamfar Saeed, Samadian Hadi, Vaeez Ahmad, Ghorbani Saadegh, Ai Jafar, Sahrapeyma Hamed, Chitosan/alginate hydrogels containing Alpha-tocopherol for wound healing in rat model, *Journal of Drug Delivery Science and Technology* (2019), Accepted.

[2] Rasool A, Ata S, Islam A, Stimuli responsive biopolymer (chitosan) based blend hydrogels for wound healing application, *Carbohydrate Polymers* (2018), Accepted.

[3] Chirani N, Yahia LH, Gritsch L, Motta FL, Chirani S, Fare S, History and Applications of Hydrogels, *Journal of Biomedical Sciences*, (4) (2015).

[4] Hoare TR, Kohane DS, Hydrogels in drug delivery: Progress and challenges, *Polymer*, (49) (2008): 1993-2007.

[5] Liu Y, He W, Zhang Z, Lee B P, Recent Developments in Tough Hydrogels for Biomedical Applications, *Gels,* 4(46) (2018): review 1-30.

[6] Ghobril C., Grinstaff M, The chemistry and engineering of polymeric hydrogel adhesives for wound closure: A tutorial, *Chemical Society Reviews*, (44) (2015): 1820-1835.

[7] Nguyen Q. V., Park J. H., Lee D. S, Injectable polymeric hydrogels for the delivery of therapeutic agents: A review, *European Polymer Journal*, (72) (2015): 602-619.

[8] Matricardi P., Di Meo C., Coviello T., Hennink W. E., Alhaique F, Interpenetrating polymer networks polysaccharide hydrogels for drug delivery and tissue engineering, *Advanced Drug Delivery Reviews,* (65) (2013): 1172-1187.

[9] Hoffman, A. S, Hydrogels for biomedical applications, *Advanced Drug Delivery Reviews*, (64) (2012): 18-23.

[10] Vashist A., Vashist A., Gupta Y., Ahmad S, Recent advances in hydrogel based drug delivery systems for the human body, *Journal of Materials Chemistry B*, (2) (2014): 147-166.

[11] Li J., Mooney D. J, Designing hydrogels for controlled drug delivery, *Nature Reviews Materials*, (1) (2016): 16071.

[12] Peppas N. A., Van Blarcom D. S, Hydrogel-based biosensors and sensing devices for drug delivery, *Journal of Controlled Release,* (240) (2016): 142-150.

[13] Li L., Shi Y., Pan L., Shi Y., Yu G, Rational design and applications of conducting polymer hydrogels as electrochemical biosensors, *Journal of Materials Chemistry B*, (3) (2015): 2920-2930.

[14] Lin S., Yuk H., Zhang T., Parada G. A., Koo H., Yu C., Zhao X, Stretchable hydrogel electronics and devices, *Advanced Materials,* (28) (2016): 4497-4505.

[15] Ionov L, Hydrogel-based actuators: Possibilities and limitations, *Materials Today Journal,* (17) (2014): 494-503.

[16] Palleau E., Morales D., Dickey M. D., Velev O. D., Reversible patterning and actuation of hydrogels by electrically assisted ionoprinting, *Nature Communications* (4) (2013): 2257.

[17] Lee B. P., Konst S., Novel hydrogel actuator inspired by reversible mussel adhesive protein chemistry, *Advanced Materials*, (26) (2014): 3415–3419.

[18] Wang Z., Wang Y., Peng X., He Y., Wei L., Su W., Wu J., Cui L., Liu Z., *Photocatalytic Antibacterial Agent Incorporated Double-Network Hydrogel for Wound Healing, Colloids and Surfaces* B, (2019) Accepted.

[19] Liu H., Wang C., Li C., Qin Y., Wang Z., Yang F., Li Z., Wang J., A Functional chitosan-based hydrogel as a wound dressing and drug delivery system in the treatment of wound healing, *The Journal of RCS Advances*, (14) (2018).

[20] Jebran A F., Schleicher U., Steiner R., Wentker P., Mahfuz F., Stahl HC., Amin F M., Bogdon C., Stahl K W., Rapid Healing of Cutaneous Leishmaniasis by High-Frequency Electrocauterization and Hydrogel Wound Care with or without DAC N-055: A Randomized Controlled Phase IIa Trial in Kabul, *PLOS Neglected Tropical Diseases,* 8(2) (2014).

[21] Brunner C A., Groner R W., Carboxy-methyl-cellulose hydrogel-filled breast implants – an ideal alternative? A report of five years' experience with this device, *Canadian Journal of Plastic Surgery*, 14(3) (2006): 151-154.

[22] Moriarty N., Dowd E., Brain repair for Parkinson's disease: is the answer in the matrix?, *Neural Regeneration Research*, 13(7) (2018): 1187-1188.

[23] Hwang S J., Baek N., Park H., Park K., Hydrogels in Cancer Drug Delivery Systems, *Drug Delivery System in Cancer Therapy*, (2004): 97-115.

[24] Rajput A., Bariya A., Allam A., Othman S., Butani SB., In-situ nanostructured hydrogel of resveratrol for brain targeting: *in vitro-in vivo* characterization, *Drug Delivery and Translational Research,* 8(5) (2018):1460-1470.

[25] Albani D., Gloria A., Giordano C., Rodilossi S., Russo T., Amora U D., Tunesi M, Cigada A., Ambrosio L., Forloni G., Hydrogel-Based Nanocomposites and Mesenchymal Stem Cells: A Promising Synergistic Strategy for Neurodegenerative Disorders Therapy, *The Scientific World Journal*, (2013).

QUESTIONS BANK

CHAPTER 1

MULTIPLE CHOICE QUESTIONS (MCQ)

1. Which of the following is the correct sequential order of the phase of healing?
   a) Remodeling, inflammation, hemostasis, and repair
   b) Inflammation, hemostasis, proliferation, and maturation
   c) Hemostasis, inflammation, proliferation, and remodelling
   d) Inflammation, development, expansion, and hemostasis

   Answer (c)

2. Phase duration of proliferation
   a) Immediate
   b) Two days – 3 weeks
   c) One day – 2 weeks
   d) None of these

   Answer (b)

3. Remodeling is the ....of wound healing
   a) Last stage
   b) Third stage
   c) First stage
   d) All the above
   Answer (a)

4. Wound healing is ....and ....process
   a) Composite
   b) Dynamic
   c) Both (a) and (b)
   d) None of the above
   Answer (c)

5. How many types of the wound?
   a) Two types
   b) 1 type
   c) Four types
   d) Three types
   Answer (a)

Short type questions

1. Define wounds? Write down about acute and chronic injuries.
2. Explain remodeling.
3. Discuss in detail about advance dressing?
4. Write down the hemostasis?
5. Define proliferation?

Long type questions

1. Discuss in detail advanced dressing.
2. Explain different approaches to wound healing.
3. Elaborate on the phases of wound healing

Chapter 2
Multiple Choice Question (MCQ)

1. Chemical constituents present in marigold
   a) Triterpenoids
   b) Flavonoids
   c) Triterpenoids and flavonoids
   d) None of these
   Answer (c)

2. What is the mechanism of turmeric?
   a) Anti-oxidant
   b) Anti- inflammatory
   c) Anti bacterial
   d) All the above
   Answer (d)

3. Give the botanical name of neem
   a) Azadirachta Indica
   b) Ocimum sanctum
   c) Both
   d) None of these
   Answer (a)

4. Hesperidin found in ……….
   a) Citrus fruits
   b) Sweet fruits
   c) All of the above
   d) None of these
   Answer (a)

5. Full form of MPO
   a) Myeloperoxidase
   b) Myeloperoxidase
   c) Myeloperoxidase
   d) None of these
   Answer (a)

Short type question

1. What is myeloperoxidase?
2. Give the chemical constituent of aloe vera.
3. What is the mechanism of orange?
4. Define hesperidin with example.
5. Give the botanical name of gudhal and their chemical constituents.

Long type question

1. What is the role of the plant in wound healing?
2. Elaborate on the mechanism of VEGF and TGF – B
3. Discuss naringenin.

CHAPTER 3

MULTIPLE CHOICE QUESTIONS (MCQ)

1. Liposome having a range of ....
   a) 0.06-7.0
   b) 0.5-0.9
   c) 0.05-5.0
   d) 0.005-5.0
   Answer (c)

2. Nanoparticles ranging from..........
   a) 10-1000nm
   b) 100-10000nm
   c) 0.1-100nm
   d) All the above
   Answer (a)

3. Ethosomes composed of....and high concentration of.........and.........
   a) Ethanol and water, phospholipids
   b) Phospholipids, ethanol, and water
   c) Water, phospholipids, and ethanol
   d) None of these
   Answer (b)

4. Liposomes have .... Solubility
   a) Lower
   b) Higher
   c) Both (a) and (b)
   d) None
   Answer (a)

5. Liposome was first developed in England by Alec D in .... year
   a)1969
   b) 1966
   c) 1965
   d) 1961
   Answer (d)

Short type questions

1. Define a novel carrier system.
2. Describe in detail phyto- vesicles.
3. Write down the limitation of the liposome.
4. Define microspheres.
5. What are the characteristics of niosomes?

Long type questions

1. Define nanoparticles? What is the application of nanoparticles
2. Discuss transfereosomes.
3. What are the advantages and disadvantages of a novel carrier system?

CHAPTER 4
MULTIPLE CHOICE QUESTIONS (MCQ)

1. Solid lipid nanoparticles consist of .... polymer
   a) Biodegradable
   b) Non-biodegradable
   c) (a) and (b)
   d) None

2. Carbon nanotube structures are……….
    a) Cylindrical
    b) Crystalline
    c) (a) and (b)
    d) All of the above

    Answer (a)

3. Size of carbon nanotube in diameter
    a) 0.5- 4.4
    b) 0.3 – 5
    c) 0.5 – 3
    d) 0.4 – 5

    Answer (c)

4. How many methods used to prepare nanoparticles
    a) 3
    b) 4
    c) 5
    d) 1

    Answer (a)

5. Give the name of natural polymers
    a) Gelatin
    b) Albumin
    c) Alginate
    d) All of these

    Answer (d)

Short type questions

1. What are the disadvantages of nanoparticles?
2. Define nanoparticles with examples
3. What are dendrimers?

4. What are the characteristics of the tumor targeting delivery system?
5. What are the uses of nanoparticles?

Long type questions

1. What are the applications of nanoparticles in the pharmaceutical field?
2. Discuss in detail the preparation of nanoparticles
3. Explain nanotube?

CHAPTER 5
MULTIPLE CHOICE QUESTIONS (MCQ)

1. Hydrogel made up of ....polymer
   a) Hydrophobic
   b) Hydrophilic
   c) Lipophilic
   d) Both (a) and (b)

   Answer (a)

2. What are the properties of the natural hydrogel
   a) Cell adhesion
   b) Cell fusion
   c) Both (a) and (b)
   d) None

   Answer (c)

3. The hybrid hydrogel is the combination of ………polymers
    a) Natural and non--biodegradable
    b) Synthetic and semi-synthetic
    c) Natural and synthetic
    d) Natural and semi-synthetic

    Answer (c)

Short type questions

1. Define hydrogel.
2. What are the advantages of the interpenetrating network?
3. What are the properties of hydrogel?
4. Define porosity?
5. What is swelling and absorption capacity?

Long type questions

1. Enlist the classification of the hydrogel.
2. Write down the difference between the natural hydrogel and hybrid hydrogel
3. Describe the theory of elasticity?

About the Authors

Dr. Balram Ambade
Associate Professor
Dept. of Chemistry, National Institute of Technology, Jamshedpur, Jharkhand, India

Prof. Balram Ambade was born June 11, 1981 in Rajnandgaon, Chhattisgarh, India. He has completed his Ph.D. from Pt. Ravishankar Shukla University Raipur in 2010 in the area of Environmental & Atmospheric Chemistry. After completing his Ph.D. thesis, he immediately started as a teaching in various reputed Engineering Colleges in India. He visited Finland for his further research. He has published 2 books and 50 research papers in reputed publications.

Dr. Rajendra Kumar Jangde
Assistant Professor
University Institute of pharmacy, Pt. Ravishankar Shukla University, Raipur (C.G.), India

Dr. Rajendra Kumar Jangde is working as Assistant Professor, University Institute of Pharmacy, Pt. Ravishankar Shukla University

Raipur (C.G.). He has completed his M. Pharma and Ph.D. from Pt. Ravishankar Shukla University (Raipur), Chhattisgarh. He is Registered Pharmacist in Chhattisgarh State Pharmacy Council, Reg. No. 668 and Life time membership of (Association of Pharmaceutical Teachers of India) APTI,CG/LM – 088

Sulekha Khute
University Institute of pharmacy, Pt. Ravishankar Shukla University, Raipur (C.G.), India

Sulekha Khute has completed her M. Pharm from S.L.T. Institute of Pharmaceutical science, Guru Ghasidas Central University Bilaspur (2016) and B. Pharm: S.L.T. Institute of Pharmaceutical science, Guru Ghasidas Central University Bilaspur.

INDEX

I

L

M

N

O

P